From Gol   to Ocean

Edited by Zoë McIntosh

Published by
Chipmunkapublishing
PO Box 6872
Brentwood
Essex CM13 1ZT
United Kingdom

First edition, October 2005

A record of this book is in the British Library

ISBN 1 904697-69-0

http://www.chipmunkapublishing.com

Acknowledgements

This book has been made possible by the help and support of many. In particular, thanks go to Rethink whose financial support helped ease the way and to Debbie and Dick for encouragement with idea in the first place and continuing support.

Special thanks go to the Rothero family for providing shelter from the storm on numerous occasions.

Thanks also to;

Sharon, whose help with the typing meant that I could worry about other things.

All at Gemini who put up with my (often) distracted presence for several years.

Richard for help and enthusiasm way beyond the call of duty.

Matthew, for a kick-start and help with the editing process.

Jen, for advice and support on demand.

Jon; partner-in-crime and comedy - here's to caffeine and crosswords.

Kate, for not giving up, and too many other things to mention. This is your book too. Thank you.

Contents

Foreword

All they taught you at school was how to be a good worker
The system has failed you,
Don't fail yourself - **BILLY BRAGG 'To Have and To Have Not'**

Three years ago I was fresh from a three month stay in a psychiatric hospital, due to clinical depression. Towards the end of my stay in hospital I had started to read (something which is notoriously difficult to do when undergoing any kind of mental confusion) and I seemed unable to stop. I devoured books about people recovering; from alcoholism, bi-polar disorder and schizophrenia, as if they were the tranquillizers that I was becoming addicted to. These were books about people suffering but more importantly, they were books about people getting better. I needed these books, these stories, almost more than I needed anything the hospital provided. They made me feel less like the only person to have experienced the despair and suffering that comes with these illnesses. Intellectually you might know that you not alone and you can find suffering in most places if you look for it. In a psychiatric ward you don't have to look far. But you can't really see it because at the time you don't see at all, you just feel. Feel the most gut wrenching pain that by its' very nature blinds you to others' suffering. Sometimes it just seems easier reading about it. This, at least, was my experience. As I lay there in my bed I would become the characters in the books that I was reading and I would be the one battling to gain control of my demons. These books gave me hope. And I desperately needed hope. And faith. To me the two are entwined; if you have one you must surely have the other. I see them spinning alongside me other promising better times ahead.

When I was ready and after I left hospital, I remembered these books and the message of the pages which had shown me that a life worth waking up in the morning for, was a viable option. I decided I wanted to write my own book; to open my eyes to the people I'd shared a ward with and to look at the realities of living with a severe and enduring mental illness. How it affected people's lives, their relationships, how they coped and whether recovery was possible.

Exploring the idea of recovery meant examining my own notions of what it meant. In my dictionary, one of its' definitions was 'restoration to a former and better condition'. Not in my world. In my world and in my book I think recovery is defined by the individual. For me it means coming to an acceptance that I will never be the same person that I was before but that I will be a different one. That I will keep putting one foot in front of the other.

I also wanted to write about the universality of mental illness and in the end this proved to be easy. It can affect anyone old or young, rich or poor, black or white. It occurred to me recently that its' indiscriminate nature could be the very reason why the stigma that surrounds mental illness is still so prevalent. Perhaps the reason journalists persist in misusing the term 'schizophrenic' in their slapdash journalism, or that the image of the knife wielding schizophrenic is perpetuated, is because in this way people can remain detached. Mental illness is still something that belongs to the 'other'. A discussion or a debate about it might require the facing up to the possibility that it could be you, your partner, your brother or sister and that is just too uncomfortable. Better to remain detached.

I want to make that detachment a bit more elusive. Giving people the opportunity to talk about their illness and their lives in their own words - not recorded and analysed through the eyes of psychiatrists or other mental health professionals - allows them to be real, to go beyond the one-dimensional. With any luck slightly harder to stay detached from.

Some of the interviews in this book make uncomfortable reading but I didn't want any cleaned-up, sparkling versions of people's lives. I wanted the truth; their truth. Which does not mean to say that everything they say is true but that everything they say at times says something about them, and at other times, something about their illness. As well as what they don't say or choose not to say. The nature of interview however, means that their truth also becomes my truth if you like. I paint you a picture, but a picture with words. These are their words, their poses but ultimately I am the artist and I paint what I see. I have tried to represent how these people have appeared to me. The resulting stories are the paintings that I as the artist produced thus all were subject to my gaze. Paintings cannot tell you everything about a subject just as these stories cannot tell you everything about a person or about an illness.

Just as a picture can show a place, a time, a dimension, colours and textures so can these stories. But whilst pictures and stories stay static, people do not. These stories represent a moment in someone's life but three years is a long time and all the subjects have all moved on to other times and other dimensions. I certainly feel a long way from that hospital bed.

The hardest part about writing this book was in admitting my own hypocrisy. Coming to terms with the realisation that even at a most basic level I often do not practise what I preach. If the issue of my mental health comes up, sometimes I lie and I frequently omit or divert. I comfort myself that though I once broke my leg I don't feel the need to tell people about it, so why should I admit to the odd bout of clinical depression. I don't because I am a coward. I am not ashamed of having broken my leg but I am ashamed of having been hospitalised, of being mentally vulnerable. I can accept it in other people but I cannot accept it in myself. So I deny my experiences; lie on job forms, to new acquaintances, say I am going to the gym when in fact I am going to therapy. Despite all my principles I feel if I tell people the truth I will cease to be to them the person they know, almost that I and my identity will crumble on the spot.

That I might lose the people that I love, my job, my home. Recently I had another 'episode', I was lucky, this one was minor, it passed relatively quickly - I wasn't hospitalised – and it ended with me still standing. My closest friends who had sat with me in the night during this time were sworn to secrecy, made to tell the outside world I had a stomach bug.

Why? Because I'm still scared. Despite all I know and feel about the importance of owning your experiences and admitting who you really are, I'm still scared. The people in this book are much, much braver than me and this is their book. They let me into their homes and their lives and they made me feel welcome. They trusted me with their experiences. They accept who they are and they deal with it for better or worse. For me this book is the beginning of accepting who I really am. That I will probably always have times when I think that the world is a terrible, scary place and that I don't want to be in it. I might - god help me - end up in hospital again, I might not. The truth is that I just don't know and I find that terrifying. What I **do** know is that long as I can keep sight of the hope and faith spinning along beside me, I will keep on putting one foot in front of the other.

Zoe McIntosh 2005

Kelly

Kelly was in her thirties and she was both vibrant and gentle in her letters and phone conversations. I finally met her at her flat one very wet day in Bristol. Although nervous and somewhat fragile, she displayed a keenness to talk about her experiences in order to help and educate others. Kelly recently went to court to try and gain access to her daughter but lost the case.

The only problem is that my mum is going to read this and she's going to flip her lid. My childhood was quite interesting but I do not want to rock the boat. But it was horrific, I'll tell you that much.

I met my husband in 1990. We were both drinkers at that point. I wasn't madly in love with him, not really, but I thought the world of him. There was definitely something there. We were both working; me as a nurse, him as a builder. In February 1991 we got married. I was like twenty-four then and I thought it was about time I got married. Soon afterwards I found out I was pregnant and then we [the house] got repossessed. It was all happening. We were living in a bed & breakfast when I nearly lost my daughter on Christmas Eve. I ended up in hospital having to have lots of fluid drained off. Two months before we had Trisha we got given a flat. It was horrible. We were going to move to Portugal and so we'd sold everything – my car, the lot. So we had nothing, not a vacuum cleaner, nothing. When my daughter was born we had sod all. We didn't move in the end – I had so many problems with my pregnancy that I thought it was better to stay in England than go over to a country that maybe hasn't got the facilities. I do believe in 'meant to be'. It was meant for me to stay here; do you know what I mean? So on Good Friday my daughter was born, three days late. She weighed nine pounds. She was big!

Things were sort of up and down with his drinking. I'd taken mine in hand because I had responsibilities. I don't know if I was an alcoholic or not because I managed to give up the drink straight away. Maybe I'd just liked being his drinking partner, I don't know. But I decided that I had to take responsibility so I cut down on the drink so much and things sort of went a bit iffy. I wasn't going out drinking and I was being left at home with my daughter. When Trisha was about four months old, I managed to get a job in a community care home to earn us a bit of money, but by then I wasn't eating and I was getting unwell. I was admitted into hospital in May 1996. I'd been going to the doctor every few days; I was hallucinating a lot. I thought the Masons were after me. I was seeing things, but I was on a high as well. Totally off my trolley, really. I was only about six-and-a-half stone and I knew I wasn't right. But I quite liked not being quite right, If that makes sense. (*laughs*)

Then my husband, although we were separated at the time, came up one night, saw the state I was in and phoned the doctor. At that time he wasn't malicious or anything and I believe he was doing it for me. Anyway, the doctor came up and gave me all these tablets – tranquillisers they were. I was popping them like sweets. Next day I went into hospital. I was saying all along that I wanted my daughter put into temporary foster care, so she could have someone who knew a little bit about what was going on and could explain it to her. Instead, she was just shuttled from here to there, between my husband, my in-laws, and my mum and dad. It was absolutely fucking crazy. She was just dumped in the hospital twice. I was told to get out of there and look after her. And that's not funny. I had so much going on in my head. And I'm not the only one. There are so many mothers going through what I went through that something has to be done. I think some support is needed; the right support. It should depend on the individual. I think there is support out there, but there's not a *choice* like there is, say, with medication.

I'm off all my meds[1] now. I use alternative therapies instead and they suit me fine. I'm into crystals. Meditating, now and again like. I have reflexology because I can afford that now I'm on my DLA[2]. My meds made me worse – made me like a bloody zombie. I didn't talk, I didn't eat. They really made me quite ill. But in a funny way they saved me in the

---

[1] Medication.
[2] Disability Living Allowance.

end. Even though I lost my daughter; and I believe much of what happened with her, was to do with my medication, not because of my manic depression. I was unable to do anything. Yes, the medication had a lot to do with making me ill, not making me better. Though in the end it saved me because it made me that numb. I think if I hadn't been on it, I would have walked over a bridge or something because of all that was going on.

When I got out of hospital, I had full charge of my daughter. The divorce was put on hold because of my being ill. I am divorced now, though. I came out about July time and I wasn't really feeling better. I had to come out because my parents said they wouldn't look after my daughter any more. They thought being in hospital was like being in a holiday camp. People don't understand that when you're high it looks like you're having a good time – and you are in a way – but you're not right, and you need sorting out. People just think you're having a wonderful time. But I wasn't. Anyway I came out and I was, you know, up and down.

Trisha had regressed back to being like a baby. Right back she went and she had to have nappies again. Buggy everywhere, bottle-fed, a dummy. She was as bright as a button before that; she'd started talking in sentences really early. But by the time I came out of hospital she was like talking all baby language, which I'd never seen her do before. So I had that to contend with as well. But I wasn't in my right mind; I wasn't thinking straight and my sleeping was terrible. If she behaved like that now I'd be sensible enough to deal with it. I've always been a responsible parent, apart from when I've been ill. She wouldn't go to sleep either. That's probably because she thought I was going to disappear. It was my fault maybe, because I hadn't explained that I was going into hospital, and what all that meant, at the time. But then I didn't know what was going on myself. I think that when you're ill, there should be people around to help you, to help with the kids, to explain stuff to them. It is all a lottery and it's not on.

My ex-husband snatched her in the October. He's done it twice. The second time I didn't get her back. The first time in October ... *(pauses)* he came over after he'd had her for the weekend and an argument started, about money and everything and then he just put her in the car and took her off. But to be quite honest, I really didn't give a shit. I know that sounds awful, but at that point, even though I love her – I love my daughter to bits – it was one less thing I had to worry about. I know that sounds really, really bad. But at that time, it all just seemed to be a mess that I could not get out of. I didn't even have the energy to be suicidal. I was that fucking numb, I didn't know what to do. It wasn't ... *(pause)*.

You can't describe it. It was as if someone had taken my heart away. Part of me was gone.

I got her back that time. He never really wanted to have her. I think he just wanted to punish me. I think he was really upset that I chucked him out and everything. I think it was his way of punishing me, you know. We were both sick then. Even though his hadn't been picked up on yet, we were both very, very sick. The Christmas of that year I still wasn't eating. I think I bought Trisha two Christmas presents and that was it … *(pause)*. It was horrific. Really, really horrific. I just didn't care. Do you know what I mean? I wasn't beating her up or anything but I didn't … it was like all my energies were zapped.

Even now, I still can't do what I used to. The only way I can describe it is to say it's as if you've got a brick wall in front of you and it's like you're chipping at it with a sledgehammer, or a pickaxe, or even a teaspoon sometimes. That's it, you start chipping away with a teaspoon and you are getting nowhere, but, bit by bit you change your tools. You keep trying different tools and you do manage to chip away. To be where I am now, to be at this point, has taken me quite a few years and people have been quite nasty. Like the people who've got Trisha. Every time I've got better or have been getting better, they've stopped access. A lot of people don't understand it; it's as if they think you asked to be ill. They don't realise that it's probably because you do care about people that you've ended up ill yourself. But I've learnt a lot from my illness; I've learnt a hell of a lot because of it. I had a really bad relapse last year and I ended up in special care. I was supposed to get a phone call from the person who was looking after my daughter and I never did.

After my ex-husband had snatched my daughter the first time, I'd had a funny feeling that he was thinking about doing it again. I decided I wasn't going to let him have her for a while, but he started doing my head in. He was turning up drunk and all sorts. So two days before her fifth birthday he phoned and said, 'Oh please, please, I'd love to have her for tea and everything,' and I said, 'Well I'll ask Trisha then. I'm pissed off with this. If Trisha wants to see you then fair enough.' I went to school to pick her up and I said, 'Look, your dad wants to see you,' and she said, ' Oh, I'd like to see my daddy.' So I said, 'Right then, I'll phone him and you can go and see him.' That was the last time I had her – two days before her fifth birthday. She never came back.

I was supposed to meet him at my mother-in-law's to pick her up and I went round there, and she said, 'Tom won't let you have Trisha back.' I knew where he lived though, so I went round there and all I did was bang on the door saying 'Please let me have my daughter back.' I didn't break no windows or nothing. The window was open on the second occasion I went round there, and I got hold of this dried flower arrangement his girlfriend had on the window ledge and slung it into the room but I think most women would have gone a bit loopy-loo at that point like. I didn't fight anyone, or smash any windows, even though I felt like I could have done. Anyway, the third occasion, all I done was slap him across the face and went 'you bastard', and then went back down to my friends to finish my cup of tea. The next thing I fucking knew, there were two bloody police cars there and I was arrested. Then, because I tried to escape out of the front window, they handcuffed me. They didn't lock them properly so they went right into my wrist and really hurt, and then I got banged up for seven hours in a police cell. The psychiatrist came and I ended up in hospital, and by then I was glad. I just wanted ... *(pause)*. It just seemed to be, at that point, that I was just out of control and the whole situation was out of control and I don't know if anyone could have helped me or not, but I was just on one. I was glad I was in hospital, but then I had to go to court to try to get custody, and I lost because I was so ill and because I was in hospital. It's not only the police who are prejudiced, it's everyone. Sometimes it has been a bloody farce. Because I have this so-called mental illness stamped all over me, I've had to fight all the way. I've always stuck to being honest, though, and I think it pays off in the end. My psychiatrist and my nurse know the truth about me. Even though it would be easier sometimes for me not to tell them the truth, I've stuck to it and they're behind me. They believe me.

I've had to prove to people that I'm not as mad as a hatter. Most people know me and they know I've got a heart of gold. Everyone's got a path, and I've got well, not so much a path, as a philosophy. I've got my own philosophy in life, I'm not religious but there's a lot of things I believe in, and I call this my 'higher power'. If you go with your higher power, well then things do work out. And I believe in karma. People who have done me harm will get their comeuppance. It might not be the same way they've dished it out to me, but I do believe that what goes around comes around. I'll keep fighting.

The psychiatrist went to see my daughter recently. He's actually quite bothered about where she is now, but because they're so close, her new mam and her, he's worried about what to do for the best. So we're all having family therapy now. That's another year, and at the end of that I won't have seen my daughter for about two-and-a-half years. I haven't done anything wrong apart from being ill. But as long as it sorts my daughter out and she don't go through what I've been through then I can put up with it. I think everyone gets ill. They either get ill young and then recover, or commit suicide. Or they end up with senile dementia when they're older. I hope I've been through it young and recovered, or am recovering.

Hopefully Trisha will have a wonderful life. She'll have loads of children and she'll find a nice man. Though I hope she will look at herself and get herself sorted before going out and getting herself mixed up in all sorts of wonderful things. Because I was quite ill, really, and obviously it had an effect on her. I mean if she can get family therapy then, though that's a bad thing for a ten years old to be having and I wish she didn't have to, if it sorts her out then maybe it'll be worth it. Are you with me or not?

She's not well at the moment. She's hiding food. I don't have a contact phone number but I have an address and I send her letters now and again, but to be quite honest, I'm even giving up on that. The woman looks at them first to make sure they're all right. But I already show my nurse them anyway, before I send them, because I know what sort of evil woman she is. She might change them, so I show Jenny[3] ... *(pause).* I'm just getting pissed off. All along the line, I've said that my daughter is going to end up with mental problems, you know. I've stuck to my word even when I was really ill, and as far as I'm concerned, it's my daughter who now has to pay a heavy price. It is quite sick. That is why I'm telling you my story.

---

[3] Jenny is a CPN (Community Psychiatric Nurse).

I had a bad night last night because it really upsets me thinking about it all. I love my daughter to bits. If my story can help someone else going through what I've gone through, well, you can't put a price on it. I wouldn't do it for money or for a fancy magazine or anything. But if people can just learn something from it, then what I've gone through and my daughter has gone through hasn't been in vain. It all seems to be left until it is too fucking late. There's not enough looking at ways to stop people from getting mental health problems. And it seems to me you have all the support when you're really, really ill, but when you start getting better, or when you're on your way there, it's all taken away. It seems to be there only when you're really off your trolley. Mind you, I have a nurse, Jenny, once a fortnight now and I'm fine. I only really have her for talking through stuff about my daughter, like how it upsets me when I cannot talk to her. I like Jenny, I class her as a friend and that's important. Other mothers have helped as well. I wouldn't say it's just the mothers who understand, but there are a good network of us. A lot of men don't fully understand what it's all about, to have your child taken off you when you've done nothing wrong.

When people say, 'Have you got children?', I'll say 'yeah', but in my heart of hearts, she's gone. To look at it that way, well, that's the only way I can survive. That's why I stayed ill for so long – through the pain of missing her so

23

much. Now I've had to let her go out of my heart and that's sad, but that's the way it is. I think she's done the same. I think that's the only way she's been able to cope with it. That's why she doesn't want to see me. It's her way of coping with the situation.

I still have many hang-ups, like for instance now, at this moment, my boyfriend hasn't texted me back, so I feel a bit panicky. I've got to sit down and try to think, 'Hang on a minute, it's only a man.' That might sound awful but I've got to put things in perspective, otherwise I can start losing the plot. I have got a lot of hang-ups, but I am talking all those through with my nurse. Once I texted my boyfriend because he kept saying things like 'Do this Deb, do that Deb,' and I texted him saying, 'Sometimes it's easy to look at other people's gardens, but it's harder to actually look at your own.' And he didn't know what the fuck I was on about. He phoned me up saying, 'What are you going on about? You haven't got a bloody garden.' And I said, 'It's a spiritual garden. It's easier to look at other people's stuff and see what's wrong with them.' Many people do that, because it's less painful than actually looking at their own stuff. Whereas I'll sit down and I'll look at my own stuff. I guess that's why I'm recovering.

I work on a voluntary bus, helping old people on and off and that's really spiritual. It's a lovely bus. A woman came once to have a look round on the bus, and she enjoyed the trip so much she stayed on for two journeys. We put old music on and we've got nicknames for everybody. We all dress up at Christmas and Easter and give them a drop of wine, and we have a real laugh. Even if you feel like shit when you get on that bus, there's something about it that's so magical, you never come off feeling bad. Yeah, it really is a magical bus. *(laughs)* They've been very supportive. I think you need honesty, as well, to recover. To say you're having a bad day, not to pretend. Sometimes I go to bed for a bit and my boyfriend will come home and ask what I've been doing in the day, and I could pretend that I've been doing something else rather than going to bed, but I think, 'no', because I'm wouldn't be being honest with myself or about myself. If I need to go to sleep for an hour, I'll go to bed rather than getting really ill and tranquillized up to my eyeballs and ending up back on the ward. If that's what it takes then that's what's got to be. Have an hour, relax and that's the end of it.

I believe in hugs, you know. If someone were ill, I'd give them a hug. It's hard, because … *(pause)*. It's hard because when you're really, really at your wit's end, nobody can tell you what to do, what you should be doing. There's no point in saying, 'Oh you'll get better. Shake yourself out of it.' Do you know what I mean? It depends on each individual doing things when the time's right for them. You have to find your own point. One night I looked up and I said, 'Is anyone there? Can you please help me?'. I was just lying on my mattress, not interested in fuck-all like, really depressed. And the whole bedroom lit up and I haven't looked back since. I'm not religious, but I've got something on my side, I know I have. It's amazing. I'd died there on that mattress. I had definitely died. Then there came this turning point, this light.

I think sometimes just knowing someone is there helps. I know a few people who are having a bad time at the moment. I just think that even though they're really ill, having a sense of humour with them is very important. Like I'll say to my mate Sarah, because she's only got one leg: we'll put a record on, our favourite song, a cheer-up song, because it's important to have those songs that cheer you up. Anyway, I'll go 'Shake a leg then, Sar.' And she's got her walking stick and she'll be jigging up and down, shaking her leg. She says, 'Oh, you do cheer me up.' I think even when people are really depressed, they want to be able to see the funny side. As long as you're a bit careful of what your sense of humour's all about, humour can really break the ice. Do you know what I mean? I've proved that so many times.

One of my philosophies is that when you're having a bad day, remember that it's just that day – tomorrow could be better. Mind you, I don't always pay attention to my philosophies. *(laughs)* Sometimes I don't get it right and then I can really get on one. It's trying to remember what you *have* got, not what you haven't got. Things could be a lot worse. Think on the positive side. It's good to be able to do something nice. Have a nice bath: a lavender bath. To be able to look after yourself, to love yourself, I think that's the most important thing, because if you don't love yourself, you can't expect anyone to love you. You've got to love yourself, warts and all. It's a hard one though.

I can think about the future now; before I couldn't. Now I can see me maybe getting another car, because I've got a driving licence, and going back to work. I'd like to do something in mental health. I think I've got a lot of qualities that I think are important. Rather than thinking that what we've been through is a bad thing, I think it's important to try to think of it as a positive thing. There's so much negativity around mental illness. Perhaps it's made us nicer people. Maybe that's your path, maybe you were meant to be ill and maybe you only get given what you can handle. Sometimes things aren't always black and white are they? Sometimes they're a shade of grey.

Susan

I interviewed Susan at her flat in Bridport, Dorset. She was incredibly warm and welcoming, with a ready supply of coffee and chocolate biscuits. She was sixty-eight years old and had been diagnosed with bipolar disorder for thirty-one years. Susan enjoyed gardening, having coffee with friends and going to church, although she insisted she was 'not very devout'. I last spoke to her a few months after the birth of her second grandson, whose arrival she was slowly getting used to.

I think my mother had manic depression[4]. It was undiagnosed but she showed symptoms of being depressed for periods and high for periods. She left school when she was thirteen and both she and her sister went into the theatre. Her mother literally took them around from repertory company to repertory company. Quite extraordinary. She'd wanted to dance and was absolutely certain she was going to do ballet. Which she did until she was about fourteen and then they looked at her physically and said she was never going to be tall enough. She had - I suppose - a devastating time while she decided what she was going to do instead. The obvious thing was to go into the theatre, and she did very well in the years before she married my father.

They had me just a year after they were married. She was so determined to do the right thing that she turned

---

[3] Manic Depression is an alternative term for Bipolar Disorder.

down good jobs, which would have meant travelling away. By the time my father went away during the war she was working for the BBC. He came back when I was eight and I think they had both decided by then that their marriage was hopeless. They tried it for a couple more years until I was ten, at which point he was working in a marvellous musical in London. He was free all day and he would go down to the swimming pool, where he met his second wife. I don't think there were any rows. Anyway, I never heard or witnessed any rows or things between them. They were very restrained about the whole thing.

I was a happy child but I was different. In those days it was unusual to have parents who were divorced. It was actually a bit of a bonus for a bit. People used to invite me to tea and say, 'Oh, poor Susan', sort of thing. My father's side of the family were absolutely shocked and horrified because they were so conventional. They'd never met anyone in the theatre and never had a divorce in the family. My mother was struggling to keep me on £1 a week from my father. Even then it was a small amount. That's why we went to Australia on the £10 scheme; *(laughs)* You had to pay ten pounds, stay for at least two years and you had to be sponsored, or you'd have to pay your passage back. So we stayed for the two years. She was very homesick. I think otherwise I would have stayed and life would have been completely different perhaps, I don't know. But she felt she couldn't leave me. I loved it over there. I went to Art College, in Sydney before getting thoroughly disillusioned with it. I came home once and said to my mother, 'I don't think I'm going to do art any more. I think I'm going to be a nurse.' Upon which she nearly fell out of bed. *(laughs)* I think I'd had a premonition that my life was never going to be easy and if I was going to rely on art to support myself through it I'd end up like my parents. They were always out of work, or 'resting', as they called it, and struggling financially. I thought, 'I'm not going to let that happen to me.' Although I realised that nursing wasn't hugely well paid, it was secure. I'd never have to be without a job and I'd always have something to fall back on. I came back to England and started my training. I loved it but I was always … *(pauses)* it was hard work for me. I found that although I loved to talk to the patients, I was always worried – unnecessarily, probably – that I couldn't cope with situations. The first time I'd get to a new ward, I'd get terribly worked up and stressed. I always finished that day with a banging headache.

I think I realised even then that I wasn't coping the way most of my friends were. They were fine and would sail through it. I'm sure it wasn't because I wasn't capable. I didn't talk to anyone about it because it seemed to be almost shameful, really. It wasn't a thing you bragged about, the fact that you were terribly worried. The nightmares I used to have! The worst time was standing in the dining room before we went on night duty, waiting to be told which ward we were going to be on. I can remember my knees almost giving way - I was so frightened. I mean I was always fine when I knew where I was going but it was cruel because you'd get on to a ward, and do perhaps two nights and then you'd get moved on again. Always going through that agony. I was also not sleeping. I was just afraid that I couldn't cope with it. I was afraid I'd do something awful. I never did, but I was always afraid. I never really got over that until I was actually qualified. I then went on and did midwifery, which I absolutely adored. I was six months at Cambridge and had a wonderful summer and did all the lovely things, like May Balls and things. Then I had six months in Caversham, Reading.

It was during that time that I realised my thing was the talking bit: getting on with the patients. So I decided to do health visiting. We were given an interview – a lecture, rather – by a health visitor. I'd never heard of it until then. I loved the training, the going out and working with the health visitors and people. I did that in London, where I was at the Royal College, which was very nice. I met my future husband during that time. Then I had the added complication that although I loved the job, I was becoming all hyped up getting ready for the marriage.

I met him on a train. *(laughs)* That sounds silly. I do tend to pick up people. I can talk to anybody; it usually leads to a wonderful friendship or it gets rid of a train journey or something boring. All my life I've done this. I think I get it from my mother being an actor. Anyway, I met this chap on the train. I chatted to him quite innocently. I thought, 'Poor thing. A button missing on his Mackintosh.' He looked awfully nice. When we got off at Paddington he said, 'Can we meet again?' – as they do, you know – and I was rather thrilled. I rang a best friend and said, 'I've met the man I'm going to marry.' I knew then you see. I was sure of it. Of course, it was a disaster the whole thing. *(laughs)* I hardly knew him because he was always away. The day I met him he was going on the train to an interview somewhere in London as a merchant seaman. He was a marine engineer. Jobs were two a penny and he got it. On the strength of that job – which was comparatively well paid in those days – we decided to get married. I'd known him for three minutes. Well, three months, I'd say. *(laughs)* Yes, not much more, and he'd been away you see. I suppose I'd known him for six or eight months in total but he'd actually been away at sea for most of that time. We didn't write. Well, I would write and he wouldn't.

My mother had taken a dislike to him from the word go and she was in the background, saying, 'If you marry him, he'll ruin your life.' In fact, I had that reaction from a lot of people, but they don't tell you really, until afterwards. They could spot something that I couldn't. They could actually spot a phoney. They saw all the things that I wouldn't believe were wrong. One of the things that came out eventually was his dishonesty. I'm exceedingly honest and I'd never met anyone who wasn't and I swallowed a lot of his stories until I realised later that they were absolutely untrue. Silly little things at first, like, for instance, telling me he was two years older than I was. When I eventually saw his passport, I realised he was in fact two years younger. It wouldn't have mattered but it was the lie that bothered me – it was so petty. He didn't introduce me to his family until two weeks before the wedding. When I met them, I realised that they were absolutely ghastly and he must have been aware that I would think they were.

I got married and very quickly had Patrick. I was working too, and it was a very difficult time for me. Luckily, the daily minder was wonderful. I'm still in touch with her. As we were both earning, it meant we could afford a mortgage. We hadn't really had a home up until then: I'd gone back to mother to have the baby and then we hadn't anywhere to go. It was quite clear that mother and he loathed each other so much that we couldn't stay there. Then, because I was working, we could afford our first proper home. It was only tiny; a nice, wee home – or it could have been. By that time, I was expecting my daughter and that fitted in beautifully because I wouldn't have wanted a long gap between the children.

I was happy most of the time, except that I already knew things were wrong. Cracks were definitely starting to show. Lots of things. I thought that perhaps getting a new home would help. Then again, you see, he was away for so many months at a time that it never really gave us a chance. When I had our daughter, he was in Japan. Looking back on the marriage, which was only fifteen years – only! – he was never there when something big was happening. Like moving. I did it all. I couldn't blame him for that really, but it was a very one-sided thing. Then when he returned it was always nightmarish because he expected things to be ... *(pauses)* well, we would have to drop everything for him. He didn't understand that I was a very routine person. The children had, I hope, a very good, sensible upbringing. I don't think I would have lasted fifteen years with him had he had a shore job and been there all the time. I think it would have ended much more quickly. Even so, I did get to a solicitor when my daughter was eighteen months old, and changed my mind. I did it again when we had just arrived in Dorset, so the children were about six or seven then. I didn't leave but I got the papers drawn up and went to the solicitors. It was the third time that I eventually escaped him. He was very violent you see and he was drunk a lot of the time. He nearly killed me three times. Once I actually went to a refuge in Bournemouth with the children. Nobody but the bank manager knew where I was. Even my mother couldn't know. We stayed there for a while and then a friend looked after us. That was wonderful. They had a huge house. But my father, who lived nearby in Sussex, was convinced that I should go back to my husband and try again. He had no idea actually what had been going on. I hadn't told him because I hadn't wanted to upset him. I felt that he couldn't help the situation in any way. And he came to visit me in this wonderful house and said, 'I'm going to take you home now, this morning, with the children.'

He thought he was doing the right thing and put everything into his car, which was big, and drove us back to Dorset. When we arrived, the entire contents of the house had been smashed. From the piano down to my sewing machine. All the children's things. All smashed or ripped up, lying all over the flagstone floor. My father … he didn't know what to say. I mean he was so distraught. I can't remember what he said, even. Words to the effect that he felt he had obviously done the wrong thing to bring us back. Then my husband appeared looking very sheepish and he and my father had a long conversation. He had been physically violent to me before and of course, it all came out then. I had to tell my father. Then he went back to his wife, having had a conversation with my husband that actually ended up with, 'I trust you, as a gentleman, that you don't lay a finger on my daughter and grandchildren and that you get something sorted out.' Of course, it all began again the moment my father had left.

He never hit the children; it was always just me. The actual turning point was when I had to call the police. He was taken away and I had an injunction taken out against him. He was forbidden to come back to where I was living. At all. I think it was probably the best day of my life. At that point, I knew we were losing the cottage because he'd been paying, or rather *not* paying, the mortgage. I knew that we were going to be homeless, but he'd gone so that was OK. Almost simultaneously, the bailiffs were banging on the door. Eventually we were housed by the Council. That was another gorgeous day of my life because I hadn't had a proper home before. At least, one that I wasn't worried about losing.

I was suicidal after Kate was born. Well, not immediately after. It was more like about eighteen months and I don't think it was classed as postnatal depression. I was almost at rock bottom then and I was almost entirely dependent on telephone calls to the Samaritans. I seem to remember thinking that nobody understood. I couldn't talk to my mother, even though she was concerned for me. Obviously she knew that there was something wrong but she was always terrified of having responsibility for the children. I don't think she was worried enough to be able to say 'You get better while I have the children for a couple of months.' She couldn't do that. She couldn't bear the responsibility of two children. They were actually very easy children, not at all naughty. So I had six lots of ECT[5] while I was at home. I had them in the morning as an outpatient and went home at lunchtimes. The home help went out of the front door and I went in.It was an absolute nightmare because I was very forgetful when I got home.

There was one time I remember we went for a walk and I had no idea where I was, what time it was, and my son, who was then about four, brought me home. We were miles away on the Downs or somewhere ridiculous and it was an appalling situation that ought never to have happened. I didn't improve much after that. On the second course of ECT, I was an inpatient. In the end, my mother did have the children but she always had this thing about her: that she was still hoping to work, as an actor. She thought she might have been called for an audition and it would have been difficult with the children there. I don't think she ever was, but that was always her worry.

I was on an awful lot of drugs after that second batch of ECT. Looking back now, I ought to have had much more supervision. I was taking these pills with good intent. I

---

[4] Electro Convulsive Therapy.

mean, I was trying to keep to a routine, but I got so muddled and confused on them. I wasn't coping then at all. Fortunately, the children were four and six, so they weren't babies. The home and everything went to pot. It was terrible. It was at that point when I was at my most muddled, having terrific highs, terrific lows and all higgledy-piggledy. There was no set pattern to it. At that time, I was in this little town with two children, and I don't know what I was then – high, depressed, everything, anything. Just very ill. It was so lucky that my new GP referred me almost immediately to a psychiatrist. I'd never had a psychiatrist 'proper' before. He was wonderful and I was with him until he retired. He got me onto Lithium. My life began then. My husband was out of the way, and we got a three-bedroomed house near the children's school. They went to a good school. I should have been happy then but unfortunately, there were still these waves, these moods. Sometimes there's no reason.

I had quite a long period when I was working properly. Years, in fact, working well and happily. The main part of that was working on district[6]. This suited me much better. Visits had to be done but I was probably more relaxed because I was more on my own, driving a car between visits, and knowing each patient quite well. Of all the years of my nursing, I enjoyed that the most. However, I'd started to drink at that point. I'd actually began to do it

---

[5] Susan refers here to her time as a District Nurse.

towards the end of the marriage. He was always drunk, always going out and coming in late. I thought that as I was trying to make a go of it, I could go out with him in the evenings, and he wouldn't drink so much because I was there. It was quite ridiculous of course, because we both ended up drunk. I began to drink more and more. Then, after he'd finally gone, I was still drinking. I was terribly ashamed of it and so I was drinking at home. In my book, women don't go into pubs and drink alone. We just don't, even now - unless we're drunkards. I wouldn't be seen in a pub, and at the time, I had a certain status because I was driving around in a uniform. I knew I shouldn't be drinking, and it was a very bad time. It got out of hand. Eventually I stopped working, not because of that exactly but because I had to have my arthritic hip replaced. I was only fifty-two but I decided the best thing to do then was to retire. I had so many things going on and I was still drinking. I told everybody it was because of my hip, which it was sort of, but I knew it was also because my drinking was out of order.

Both my children had gone when they were sixteen. Patrick went to France and then to Germany. I saw very little of him although he was always in touch. Telephone-wise he was good. Kate went up to London and again she was marvellous. She was very independent and found lots of different jobs. Eventually she went to art school but not until she was twenty-seven. That period when I was drinking, I'd given up my job and I was living alone … *(pauses)* I expect I was lonely. I really was drinking quite badly. I decided that I couldn't afford to keep a three-bedroomed house; that it wasn't fair to be on my own when so many families needed a home. I had a choice of putting in for a transfer for somewhere smaller or taking in lodgers. My mother had lodgers during the war and it could be fun or it could be awful. I decided to try it and got two from the Friary[7]. One was pretty awful. Took my chequebook. At least took a cheque and didn't come back. The other, Tony, stayed with me for nineteen years.

I knew I had to stop drinking. I was on Lithium at the time as well and I don't know if that made things even worse. I'd been to AA and to all the usual channels. I have a strange bit in my personality though, whereby if I decide to do something, I can do it. And I just sat up in bed one day and thought, 'I want to keep Tony here.' I felt responsible for him. He'd been so much better than the other lodgers might have been. He wanted to drink too and I knew I couldn't tell him not to drink and do it myself. I literally stopped. There and then. I mean I didn't give it up without a lot of difficulty. It caused a lot of problems. When I went to AA and all that, I thought they were silly old fools. I was very sceptical. When I did stop drinking, I realised that so much of what they'd said,

---

[7] The Friary was a monastery local to Susan that provided short-term accommodation to the homeless.

at the meetings, for example, had been sensible. Somehow, they had got under my skin. Anyway, I gave up and I amazed my doctors and myself.

Then my son died. He'd come over a couple of times a year from Germany. Each time, he was ... *(pause)*. He was a most charming person. He had a tremendous personality and he was awfully nice. He and I always got on terribly well. Far better than I have ever got on with my daughter. When he came home he was sometimes a bit edgy and a bit aggressive and a bit sort of 'shrug your shoulders' and go out sort of thing. Which he would never have done before but I didn't really think anything of it at the time. Drugs didn't occur to me. Looking back it now, it seems obvious. On the last but one holiday he had with us, Tony became suspicious. My son went out one day and we knew he'd be out for a long time so we searched his bedroom. We found nothing. Tony had had experiences of that sort of set-up and knew where to look. We looked in the cistern, in the loo; all the obvious and unobvious places.

By then I was almost certain that he was on drugs and I told my daughter. She got hold of my ex-husband and he went to Germany. When he came back, he said, 'Nothing wrong with Patrick. I've seen him in the bath and there are no marks on him. He's perfectly all right.' Two weeks later, he was dead. On the death certificate it said 'heroin overdose'. It was the most tremendous shock. We'll never know quite what it was. They've said it was an overdose, but we don't know the cause. We don't know whether it was bad heroin or whether it was … *(pause),* I mean the most unlikely thing is that it was intentional … but we'll never know. I've tried going through the German Embassy and they weren't at all helpful.

Kate and I flew over for the funeral and it was miserable. I came straight back while she stayed to sort out Patrick's flat. My ex-husband was there, claiming things like Patrick's leather jacket, and saying, 'I think I'll take his watch.' Anyway, I wasn't there. I couldn't have stood it. One of my first thoughts when it happened was to thank goodness my mother had died first, because she absolutely worshipped him and I don't know if *I* could have coped with *her*. Kate was devastated. She had to cope with me, as well, and this is where they say I pushed it all underneath. I didn't. I couldn't weep with Kate. I knew how upset she was and I couldn't make it worse for her. Tony was also deeply upset because he considered Patrick to be like a brother.

I think people wondered if I was even bothered. I wondered sometimes. You hear of these things happening and you imagine weeping, howling, wailing. I didn't do that and I think that was an awful thing. I never have actually really given in and cried. I've thought about it alot. Patrick's death, I mean. Perhaps more of late. I've brought it to the surface. Before I almost shoved it underneath. I didn't do anything odd. I mean, I kept all his photographs and sometimes I look at them. The only thing I can't do still is to read a pile of letters I'd sent him that Kate rescued for me, from his flat. It looks like he kept every single one. I don't know, I haven't checked. They're all in a box in that drawer over there. It's the only thing I can't do: read them. I suppose I will one day. I was stable for a time afterwards, but in 2001, I became ill again. I'd come off the Lithium all of a sudden because they decided that my kidneys were damaged. Apparently, the only alternative they had was to put me on to an anti-epileptic drug.

During that year, I got more and more depressed and so I was put on another drug to counteract the depression. For some reason, there was a mistake with it and nobody knows why. It could have been the chemist. I'm sure it wasn't my psychiatrist. Anyway, somewhere along the line I wasn't getting a full dose. I got half a dose and I wasn't well enough to notice the labels on the packets. Whether I wouldn't have gone right down if I'd had the right amount I don't know, but I went crashing. I saw the psychiatrist once or twice during that time. I was feeling so low that I couldn't even speak. Later he said he hadn't recognised how depressed I was at the time and he actually apologised to me, which was very comforting to me, coming from somebody in his position. I put him even higher on my list than he was already. I got lower and lower and lower until I was, by that time, almost completely unable to look after Tony. I managed to cook a meal five minutes before he got home, tell him I'd already had mine and go back to bed. I spent all of my time in bed. I wasn't looking after myself at all. It was so rapid; it was most extraordinary. I was hoarding my sleeping pills. I took around two months' worth. I took them with every intention. When I eventually woke up that evening, I was in hospital. The most extraordinary thing was that Tony, who I thought had gone to work, came back and found me. He only worked a couple of days a week and I'd got muddled up and got the days wrong. I hadn't expected him back until the evening, by which time I thought everything would have happened. Yes, he came back. Called up to see if I wanted some coffee, and of course I didn't answer. Extraordinary that he came back, isn't it?

I suppose I was admitted via the general hospital in Dorchester. I don't remember anything really. I woke up that afternoon on a ward that was sort of locked up, you know. They kept asking me questions, giving me questionnaires. 'How did I feel now?' 'Did I really want to do it?' For a week I was so angry. I couldn't believe that I hadn't done it, that it hadn't worked. I don't think they even gave me a washout. In other words, I just hadn't given myself enough. Or I've got a constitution like an ox. They transferred me to another unit, a sort of halfway house. It was marvellous. It was like a little hotel, it was so comfortable and there was almost one-to-one staffing. Always someone to talk to. It was probably someone to talk to that I'd needed more than anything. I think so; it's all a bit hazy. What I do remember clearly is that during that time my grandson was born. In Newcastle, and there was a great sort of fuss waiting for the phone message and everything. I was over the moon. I remember thinking, 'What was I thinking three months ago? I wouldn't have known about this if I'd ... ' *(pause)*. I'd known he was a boy when I did do it actually, because they'd had a scan.

I can't really remember what I felt about him. I met him for the first time when he was six months old and I had no gush of grandmotherly feelings. I've been through a very funny time about him and I wonder if it is anything to do with Patrick. I've only seen him about four times in all and at first, I didn't want to touch him. My daughter sensed it. She said, 'You do love this baby? You do love him don't you?' And I said, 'Of course I do.' I'm a good actor but I didn't want to touch him. Maybe it was because I didn't see him at birth. My poor daughter went through absolute hell when he was born, and after the delivery, he nearly died of dehydration. In Newcastle Hospital. That's another story though. My daughter and I have ridiculous arguments, which I know mothers and daughters do have. One of the things that nearly finished us was when she said she couldn't forgive

45

me for not being with her when John was born. That really hurt. It was something that I couldn't believe she'd said. I'd been so ill at the time. She probably didn't mean it like that. She probably meant she couldn't forget I wasn't there, full stop. A statement said in a temper. I wrote a letter to her at the time and didn't post it. I'm always doing that. It gets things off my chest. If I do write her a letter, she doesn't respond anyway. We never finish arguments. She has accepted though - and I've accepted - that we do argue. Sometimes with venom. Writing gets it off my chest. John is gorgeous. I'm very proud of him. He's a dear little chap. Last time I saw him the grandmotherly feelings did come. Just a little bit. Yes, this time they did a bit. He got up on my knee.

Richard

Richard was sixty-seven years old when I interviewed him. He had been given a diagnosis of psychosis following alcohol and drug addiction. At the time of the interview, he had been abstinent from alcohol for twenty-one years and off drugs for six. He was regularly attending AA meetings. He was a friendly, outgoing man, who laughed frequently and was clearly at ease with the whole interview process. Richard died from chronic cardiac failure on 24 February 2003.

I was born in 1946 into a family of five brothers and two sisters. My father used to drink a lot. He used to drink at the weekends and then he could become very violent. I can remember even in my early years, as a kid, the police coming up and me holding the policewoman's hand, and going under the table hiding. In our house, there was always a tense atmosphere; one that you could cut with a knife. Nobody talked about anything. I never saw my mum and dad kiss each other, cuddle or anything like that. They were always vying for our love and affection. I found it very difficult and always went more with my mother. My father never had much to do with me and I wondered why. I never thought that I was his kid. I always thought that I might have been the butcher's or the dustman's or something like that. Even from when I was very little, I felt different, alienated.

I remember me and my brothers going out playing and we were always the last ones to go in at night, when it was nearly dark. We'd stay out all day playing in the woods and everything. It was great. Indoors it was a different kettle of fish. Father's word went. There was fear everywhere. In school, my attention span was useless. I found it very difficult to concentrate and maths especially was very difficult for me. I was in classes of thirty, and I needed maths explaining to me. But they didn't have the time and if you didn't pick it up you were just left behind. So I always came last in maths. The only thing I was really good at was geography. I always came top in geography. But later on, I hardly ever went to school. I'd go in, be registered and just walk out. *(laughs)*

When I left school, I didn't know what I wanted to do. I find it's been like that all my life. I've always known what I've not wanted to do but I've never known what I have wanted to do. That's still with me today. But I've accepted it. As I've accepted most of my other shortcomings, bad points, good points, in-between points. My mental illness, my alcoholism, my drug addiction. As I've accepted all that, I've accepted me more. By accepting whom you are and what you are, you can have a more peaceful life, a more productive life. Because … *(pause)* you know what's going on. You know what's going on with yourself. I must have had about thirty jobs in all. None of which I ever stuck at. I had three jobs in one day in the Sixties. *(laughs)* Start in the morning, chuck the job in. Go round somewhere else, down the road onto another building site. Start the same day there and then. Chuck it in. Go to another building site or an old factory and get a start for the next day. In the Sixties, you could do that.

I found the building trade suited me down to the ground. I loved getting mucky. It was a hard man's sport, if you know what I mean. They were heavy drinkers. I got into the drinking game through that, really. I drank heavily straight away. But drink never really suited me. I was sick quite often through drinking, but I persevered at it. Drink gave me a release from myself. I used to get anxious very easily. I found it very difficult talking to members of the opposite sex. I used to go red at the drop of a hat. I would get tongue-tied very easily. I found conversation difficult. Communication was difficult. I found life hard – very, very hard work. I treated drink as a panacea for all my ills. I was like a leaf in the gutter just being blown about by circumstances. I stopped giving my mother and father money for board because most of my money was going on drink. I expected them to keep me for nothing. I had no sense of responsibility whatsoever. No sense at all.

The first serious girlfriend and the first sexual stuff that I had was when I was seventeen. I met a girl in the pub. I was on a pinball machine and there was two girls sitting down. One of my mates was sitting with one of the girls and when I went out to the loo he follows me in there. He says, 'You know those two girls that I'm sitting with? One of them fancies you.' I thought she was roughly the same age as me. She was good-looking, had a miniskirt on, all the business she was. 'Whee!' I said, 'Does one fancy me?' I couldn't believe it. I couldn't believe that anyone would like me. I didn't think that anyone could (long pause) ... So I went out with her and we had sex. The first time was in her back shed. We were both drunk, both of us, and we woke up in the morning together. Locked together in each other's arms. *(laughs)* Locked together. (*claps*) It was about half-past six in the morning. A summer's morning. And I had to get on a bus home. I was drunk. Everything happened when I was drunk. I courted her in pubs really. One day I came in from work and her father was sat there talking to my father and mother. My dad says to me, 'Do you know how old Christine is?' I was seventeen. I said, 'No I don't,' but by then I did. He said, 'She's fourteen.'

The police got involved because she became pregnant, after I'd been going with her for about six months, something like that, maybe a year. I went down and saw the detectives after they'd interviewed her. They interviewed me and they said, 'No action will be taken against you. She says you're not the first man she's had sex with. She's had two or three people.' Yeah, I found that out as well. She wasn't Snow White or anything but I was in love with her. I thought the world of her and she thought the world of me. We really did but I think it was based on sex. I did what I used to do to everybody: give all my love and expect all love back. I used to put all my emotional eggs into her hands and say, 'You love me back the same.' I was asking too much of people in relationships. No eggs back in my basket for me. But I loved her. We got married in a registry office after she'd had the baby. She had Colin. I had a son. He's thirty-five now and he suffers from schizophrenia. Mental illness runs in the family. He was diagnosed when he was about twenty. I could see it coming. He was so gentle and kind, loving and everything. But he couldn't handle life. I knew he couldn't.

So I'd got married. And do you know what I thought on my wedding day? I thought, 'What have I done? I've done it now.' We lived with my parents at first. My relationship with my parents was strained and everything, but I was trying to buckle down and do the best I could. My drinking was curtailed just to weekends. I didn't take my wife out much. I expected her just to do the business, look after the baby and stuff like that. Eventually we got a place of our own and she became pregnant again about two years later. We had Robert. So we had two kids. We were on a losing horse straight away, we were so immature ourselves. I was working all right, trying my best to pay the rent regularly, giving her enough money to get food in. But my drinking was increasing and all of my spare money went on drink. I hadn't touched any drugs by then. I looked at drug addicts who stuck needles in themselves and I thought that'd be the lowest of the low. I'm a hard man. I was a hard man.

Being a father used to get on my nerves. The children got in my way. The crying and stuff like that. Sometimes I'd put them out in the hall, shut the door, just didn't want anything to do with them. Leave them in their pen crying. Terrible thing to do. Now I think about it, I should've changed their nappy, cuddled 'em, picked 'em up. But they were getting in my way. I was so immature. I wasn't a good father at all. I wasn't. Along came another baby, my daughter, and she was really noisy. I can remember her being really noisy and she'd stand up in her cot, rattle her cot and everything like that. I started taking Mondays off and drinking all day and subbing my money from my wages.

After about seven years of this … *(pause)*. It was on a Monday I think. My missus walked out. Looking back now, she was suffering from postnatal depression. I didn't realise it then. She'd just sit there doing nothing. The filthy nappies used to go up in a pile about two-foot high! We was all coming out in these spots and itching. One day she just disappeared. Just disappeared out of view. She just went and I found out she'd been having an affair. The kids, I tried to look after 'em: washed them, fed 'em, and took them to school. But these spots turned out to be scabies. Everything in the house had to be burnt. The council came up and burnt stuff. I burnt stuff. Fumigated the house. My little boy, Robert, he was ever so small. He had shocking white hair, blond; he was a beautiful boy. Lovely. I had to paint this stuff on him and he stood there screaming. I'll never forget it, He was stood there with no clothes on and I painted him with a shaving brush. That picture will always stay in my mind. Anyway, the spots all cleared up. But I couldn't look after my kids and work at the same time. It was too demanding. Running up and down ladders all day. So they got farmed out to other people. To foster homes.

I used to go and visit them. My eldest boy, Colin, was with these foster parents and he used to wet the bed and they smacked him. He told me about it. I went to them and said, 'You'll never fucking smack him again,' and picked him up and took him home with me. I knew that I couldn't look after him, so I took him up my mum and dad's. Told them the score. And they said, 'Don't worry about it boy, we'll bring him up. As long as you do your bit.' But even then my drinking was getting worse. At this time, I had a very close relationship with a man called Colin. I loved him as a friend. It was my first adult relationship with another man, and he died. He had a motorbike accident. And he died in hospital at two o'clock one morning. I found out about it the next day. That increased my drinking one hundred per cent. I couldn't handle the emotions that went with him dying. I drank to drown the emotions. I just used to blub; I'd sob in pubs about it because I missed him so much.

It all kicked off then. I brought the bed downstairs and lived in the living room. I had nothing at all upstairs. Someone offered me some speed. They gave me five blues. French blues. I took them and I felt marvellous. I'd never had a feeling like it. Because the beer was tasting like piss to me, I had to have top-shelf stuff like whisky to give me a buzz, right? So I was about twenty-four when my life became controlled by drink and drugs, which is quite late I suppose. It led to me becoming mentally unstable. I thought when I walked down the road that I was going to jump out under the wheels of lorries and get crushed. Thought I was going to go blind. Swallow my tongue. Choke myself. Or run around. Just run around, like a headless chicken. Lose me head. I used to have a lump in my throat a lot. It was anxiety. I used to get to the pub and drink and drink. When I drank those thoughts went away. I'd always said I'd never stick a needle in myself but it only took once and then I'd broken the taboo. From then on, I started fixing myself. I became very ill about this time and developed viral pneumonia. I was coughing up blood by the bucketful. I was nearly dead and had the most dreadful pain. I had viral pneumonia and they took me into hospital. I've never been in so much pain; couldn't straighten up because my stomach kept on contracting. I was in hospital for about seven weeks and I lost about two-and-a-half stone in weight. I couldn't eat to start with but I managed to get some food down me, and I swore I'd never smoke again.

I lived with my mum and dad for about five weeks. Then they kicked me out because I didn't pay my way. I used to go down the pub and spend it all, then come home drunk and cause an upset. They couldn't put up with it. My other brothers were drinking as well. They must have had a terrible time. We were all drunk, the bloody lot of us. When they kicked me out I took to sleeping in cars and under hedges. Wandering about half the night, sleeping in libraries during the day. In the winter when it was snowing, I used to go in the library and sit there in the warm. Drinking cheap bottles of wine, cider and bottles of cough medicine. I used to get something called a Benzedrex nose inhaler, which was like speed. I used to get the compact inside and cut it up into three parts. Then you could poke it at the back of your throat, drink it back and about half an hour later you were speeding. Everybody was at it. All the kids. *(laughs)* The chemists were going bonkers, telling us they weren't going to give it to us no more. We used to travel miles to get it. Once my mate saw a chemist getting a delivery and they had a big box of the stuff. My mate wrote out a cheque on the spot for it. He had the lot. He took the whole box! *(laughs)* Amazing!

To cut a long story short, I got into a bit of trouble and landed up in prison. I was given three years. What did I do? Two burglaries and I sat in a stolen car. They gave me a year for that. For sitting in a stolen vehicle! They were after my blood. It was in prison that I came to realise that I had a problem with drink. I wouldn't admit it to anyone else. Just to myself. I was talking to this bloke once in the carpenter's shop, where I was working. You have to work in prison see. He said, 'I'm an alcoholic,' and he told me about a meeting of Alcoholics Anonymous that went on in the prison. I thought, 'I don't want nothing to do with that,' so I didn't bother going, but that was sort of my introduction to it.

During the middle or late Seventies I was in and out of prison. They used to pick me up in a police car, take me over to Oxford in handcuffs and put me in prison. I used to look forward to it in a way. It was a bed. It was roof and food, so I didn't mind it, really. Sometimes I saw my kids, sometimes not. They were going to special schools, which they should never have been in, 'specially Colin. He had a good brain but they were all living in at this special school. I went over there really drunk once and showed myself up. But they loved to see me. They just loved it.

When I came to Oxford I'd been dry for a while, but within a week, I started drinking. I was a raving alco by then. I caused mayhem at the probation hostel. They had to close the place down in the end. I used to have coppers sitting on me, squashing me. I'd run around with knives. The drink and drugs made me to foam at the mouth. I used to take overdoses and I was pumped out about fifteen times. Once they had to shock me back to life. I'd been fighting with the porters at the hospital. I was as drunk as a Lord! They threw me down and I landed on me back; all the drink came up and I breathed it in. Someone noticed that I'd turned all blue. My heart was all over the place. They got the jump leads on me and got me going. I woke up in Intensive Care. My chest hurt me so much. I didn't know whether I wanted to live or die. I wanted to die and I wanted to live. I wanted help. *Desperately*. But I didn't know how to ask for it.

I ended up in a dry hostel, with all the down-and-outs. I was one of them. I lived there and had periods of dryness. But I went on a binge and went into alcoholic psychosis. I thought people were following me. There were film cameras out there. There were skulls grinning at me. Everything. I saw the devil. The room went jet black and then it went pure gold and I saw Jesus Christ standing in front of me. All sorts of weird things. This went on all through the night. I didn't get any sleep. I went running the next day. Running round Oxford. It was sunny. I never had no shoes or socks on. No top. Just jeans. There was crying out in the background, these workers trying to help me, but I never took no notice. In the end I got picked up by the police. They took me to the acute psychiatric ward for people who have mental confusion. I was in this room and I looked out and there were all these policemen. They had rifles and they were all firing these bullets, I felt the bullets going through me. That was really weird. There were pictures on the wall and I kept taking these pictures down and spitting where I'd taken the pictures down. People kept coming in and out of the door, bringing me a cup of tea, stuff like that. They asked me my name, how old I was, I was very confused.

It was in there that I started to get better. Until then I'd hung on to this thing called control. I'd wanted to control everything all my life. Everything that I felt. Everything. It was like hanging on to the edge of a cliff. I was hanging on and hanging on for my dear life. And I couldn't let go because I was so frightened of what was over the edge. The fear was terrifying. All of a sudden, I said these words: 'I give up.' I slumped on a table. I felt something go through my body, up through my shoulders and out of me. It was like a release from this - whatever it was - and I seemed to quieten down. I knew that everything would be all right from then on. Just in that split second. Because I'd stopped fighting everything. I surrendered and that was the key to my recovery. Surrendering. In most things in life, people say you have to fight and overcome. With alcoholism, and I would say with most things you have to surrender. Surrender and give up the fight. From there they took me to psychiatric hospital. I was in there over Easter. Because it was Good Friday, it happened to me. On a Good Friday … *(pauses)*.

I was walking round in their cell, still having the DTs [8]. I was in this cell and outside there was a clear blue sky. I got a chair and looked out at the sun. I looked at the sky and I could see rockets going from Russia to America. Passing each other in the sunlight. But I *knew* they were my deepest fears and I could rationalise it. Sitting outside of my room was this bloke reading a book. I was on twenty-four-hour watch, you see, but I didn't know that. I thought, 'What's he doing there watching me?' *(laughs)* I was paranoid, you see. I kept poking my head round, looking at him, thinking, 'What's he doing?'.

They had said to me previously, at the alcohol unit, that they couldn't help me no more. That I was a hopeless case. They said, 'We've tried everything with you and it doesn't work.' This time I said to one of the therapists, 'Can you give me one more chance?'. He says, 'Come on, Dick, we've done everything we can.' But he came back the next day and said, 'We'll give you one more chance.' I took it like a dog with a bone. I went for it and had eight weeks of group therapy. I got eye-to-eye contact and told people things I'd never told anyone else. I got honest with myself, for the first time. I became truthful. Stopped lying. Stopped covering up.

---

[6] Delirium Tremens: shaking brought on by heavy drinking.

Started saying how I really felt. Started to get in touch with my feelings. During that time, I used to see the people coming to AA meetings, driving up in cars and stuff like that. I used to think, 'They can't be alcoholics.' I was a down and out. How could they have cars and stuff like that? Course, I didn't realise that some of them had been sober for a long time and got their lives back together.

I went to my first AA meeting because after being sober for five months, without a drink, I thought, 'I don't want to drink any more. Period. For the rest of my life.' So I went to my first meeting. I went there with an open mind. A lot of anxiety was still there – sweaty hands, stuff like that; feelings of paranoia. But it was going. I went there and I identified with people, and I loved the meeting. I just fell in love with it. I got involved very heavily in Alcoholics Anonymous. It was the openness and honesty of the other alcoholics in the group and the identification with them that helped me recover. It's based on psychiatry, and philosophy and spirituality in recovery. Alcoholism is a threefold illness you see: it's physical, mental and spiritual. Many people forget that as people, we are spiritual, physical and mental beings. Often we forget the spiritual side of our lives and just deal with the physical and the mental. That drew me to it even more. I knew that when I surrendered, when I gave up, something odd had happened to me. It was strange. It was out of the ordinary. I put that down to a spiritual experience.

That's what I put it down to. I went to the library and I read every book I could. I got books on Buddhism, Taoism, I got everything that I could and read it all. I was searching for God, if you like. But he'd already got me. He'd already got me anyway. *(laughs)* I started being invited to talk at other meetings. Making friends for the first time in my life. Real friends. Speaking to people without the aid of any chemicals. Without booze, anything. It was like being reborn. It was like a new life to me. The first spring that I went through, I noticed shades of colour that I've never noticed them before. Ever. I'd just never noticed before. And it was like … it wasn't getting back my old life, because my old life was crap anyway. Before I even picked up a drink, it was bad. Bad enough anyway. But it was like having a new life. I mean, a brand new life.

I was having relationships with women. I fell in love with one. Deeply in love. We broke up because she was a lesbian. It just broke me heart. I cried and I couldn't handle it. I just couldn't handle it. I went back to my old ways, I suppose, of trying to handle it with drugs. In the end, I had psychosis again. It was awful, terrible. I had people following me. The police were following me, the DHSS was following me. All people in authority were following me. People wanted to kill me. Everything. It was so real to me. The flat I was living in was just filthy dirty. I didn't clean it. Couldn't clean it. I couldn't sleep in the bedroom because I thought the place was haunted. I woke up one night and there was all these figures dancing round the bed. It was evil stuff. I just went off my head. My doctor put me in an acute ward. I stayed in three-and-a-half months. They diagnosed me as having paranoid schizophrenia, brought on by an overdose of amphetamines. They said, 'That's your diagnosis and I'm afraid that's what you've got to put up with now.' I said, 'OK, I accept that.' They said I had it for life. But I've recovered from it a lot. I started getting better, slowly but surely. Staying away from alcohol – I never picked up a drink again. Once I went to pick a drink up, and I pulled my hand back. I had been fifteen years sober then. I knew that if I picked a drink up I'd be dead within a fortnight. I'd be dead. Gone. Plus, I didn't have enough money to have a good session. *(laughs)* So I didn't pick it up and I slowly recovered.

I cope with being not well by not keeping it a secret, by talking about it; because there's a great saying in life, which I stand by: 'You're as sick as your secrets,' right? That applies to anybody in life. When I'm not well, I think people are following me. I'm not very well at the moment actually. I don't mean physically, I mean mentally. I think that there's people living opposite me, who are watching me from their balcony with binoculars. I wave at them sometimes. *(laughs)* I think that the television has a camera in it. When it's cooling down or warming up it clicks and makes noises. I go; 'Good morning' or 'Good afternoon'. But I know that it's my

illness making me think those things. I know that. And I can
... I can rationalise that. I don't switch the telly off. I don't let
it control me at all. I don't let it have its way with me. I don't
have that. I won't have it. I won't let it control my life at all.
What happens is, I phone a friend and talk about it. Talking
about it brings it out in the open. Anything that you hide, that
you keep back, makes you sicker and sicker. If you bring a
thing out into the open, into the light, then it takes away its
power. It takes away its power over you, so that you can
overcome it by surrendering. I try to be light-hearted about it.
I pray about it. And as I said, I talk about it. I meditate on it. I
have books and things that I use. I go to church every
Sunday. I started doing that about three years ago and this
is what helps me get over my illness and my difficulties. My
faith in God, right?

I went to church and got baptized and there were
about eight or nine of my mates, all blokes, right, all hard
men, yeah? You wouldn't have believed it if you'd said to me
a few years ago that I'd be in a church with all my brothers
and mates. Watching me get baptized. Pouring water over
my head. We done that and then about nine months – or
maybe six months – later, I got confirmed by the Bishop of
Oxford. There was singing. The church was packed, there
was flowers everywhere, it was a wonderful night. All my
relatives came from everywhere and all the children's
relatives, mothers, fathers, uncles, aunts, sisters and

brothers. And the singing. Everybody was singing and it was lovely. I got a great, great lift from it.

A classic thing that happened to me recently was that I cut down my tablets. They made me feel a bit dopey and I thought they was causing me my weight problem. My 'fatism' as I call it. But I cut down and I got so depressed. The depression was awful and I just couldn't see a way out of it. I went to see my psychiatrist, who I don't think much of to tell you the truth. She looked at my prescription and said, 'Oh, you need more than that,' and she doubled my dose, so it was twice as high as it had been before I cut down. What happened was, I took this medication and I got up to have a piddle and I was staggering everywhere. Like a drunk man. My co-ordination was gone, right? I pissed myself and everything. And I couldn't remember things. I woke up on top of the bed. I went to put my trainers on and I'd pissed in them as well for some reason. I didn't know how it had happened. So I decided to come down to what I'm on now. And I take that and it suits me. I get a good night's rest. What it did was take away the depression. I know that I'm a depressive as well as a schizophrenic you see. My friend said to me, 'Dick, you're more a depressive than you are a schizophrenic.' He said, 'You ain't like them others, you're different from them. You don't strike me as being ill like them.' I said, 'I am.' I said, 'I am ill and I do suffer. I suffer.' But what I do is I've got a way of dealing with it, what they

64

ain't got. I've got it under control. Yeah, I've got it under control.

Andy

Andy was a smartly dressed, self-effacing man. He overcame his natural shyness to talk about his experiences because he believes that in order to reduce its stigma, mental illness needs to be discussed. He is married and has a daughter.

I joined the Navy in 1979. I went all round the world on a ship. Went to America for three months and was based in Gibraltar for a year. It was great! I made friends in the Navy. I had good friendships. You have to get on with people. You learn to get on with them because you're close together. You kind of build up friendships and go out socialising and there's quite a lot of drinking involved. Then in 1982 I was on leave and I got a phone call saying 'The Argentinians have invaded the Falklands, come back to your ship.' I was about nineteen. Quite young really.

I was working on an aircraft carrier, the HMS Hermes, which was the flagship *(pauses)*. It's a bit disjointed this, just coming out when I remember it. Coming out of Portsmouth it was nice to see all the crowds seeing us off, you know, out of Portsmouth Harbour. Anyway, you'd do your six hour watch and then had six hours off when you'd wash and clean your clothes. So you didn't get much sleep really. We did this day and night for about three months. When the action stations come on, everybody had to get on watch. They'd say over the tannoy, 'missiles released'.

Very bizarre. One went across our bow. We were sort of point on to the missile as it were. It aims for the biggest target. We could've easily lost the war you know.

Well anyway, a missile hit 'The Sheffield' (the destroyer). A missile went into it, when it was on our horizon. That was horrible. The injured were brought on to our ship, burning. There had been a ship design fault - the ships then were made of aluminium which burns white hot. Which was a mistake really. I've got pictures of the ships you know, when they'd been gutted by fire; that the ship's photographer took when he went up in a helicopter. The wounded and the dead were brought on to our ship because we were the nearest. The dead bodies went into the back of the ship into the ward room where the Officers were.

I was an engineer mechanic. Radio, first class. Electronics really, maintaining the electronics, that's what I did. The radar, things like that. You're just a sitting duck really. If you were a soldier in the Falklands, you've got a bit of control about where you are and what you do. But if you're on a ship and a missile hits you, there's nothing you can do. You don't know until it hits you.

I found it a strain, you know, mentally and I had a few strange thoughts. I didn't realise what was happening to me really. I had no background of mental illness. I'd started to have delusions. Can't remember them really. Through the stress and pressure, I think. I remember later on I had feelings of grandeur. Thinking I was an important person, you know something more than I really was.

I came back from the Falklands and my parents and family had a party and things like that. The war had ended. The whole war only took about three months. So when it finished we sailed back. It wasn't a very long war at all. I stayed for a little time in Portland. Then I was stationed for a year in Gibraltar where I was based on a receiver station. I found it quite difficult there. It was only six miles all the way round the island. I was away from home and I'd been having a relationship with a girl there and I left her behind. That was quite hard that was. Also it's quite insular in Gibraltar and I began to feel quite ill then. It was sort of building up and I felt quite psychotic. Without knowing it really. I didn't realise what was happening to me. I think when I was in the Falklands, I was only fleetingly ill. Just through the stress of it all. Just for a little while really. I seemed to be alright when I came back. But when I went to Gibraltar I went downhill quite a lot you know. I became quite withdrawn with it, and unhappy and upset.

And then when I came back from Gibraltar, I left friends I'd made there behind and felt quite isolated. Before you join the Navy you have friends from school and things.

But you lose touch when you join the Navy. You've then got different friends in the Navy with each draft. But when you get home there's nothing. I spent a lot of time in bed.

I went back to Portland and did Navy work. Sort of shift work. Three days on and a couple of days off. I got even worse then. I was just surviving to work. I'd go to work and then come home. I wasn't looking after myself and I thought...(*pauses*) I thought the radio was talking to me. I was completely paranoid. Like the book '1984', which funny enough was also the year I was quite ill. Sometimes I'd be happy you know in a sort of like, fantasy world, in my brain and sometimes I'd be really down and depressed.

One day I got as much paracetemol and alcohol as I could as I could and drunk as much as I could and had as many tablets as I could. I think I was very psychotic. The fact that it was a bad thing to do didn't even cross my mind. It's a terrible thing to do - what a waste of a life - but at the time it's just a way out really. I suppose it was a cry for help. You're so psychotic and it feels so horrible, what you feel inside and what's happened to you. You become more and more depressed and anxious. I had quite a lot of anxiety. You can't see a way out really. You just get more and more ill. Also, I'd put in to come out of the Navy at that time and I suppose the stress of having to cope outside and find another job just added to the problems as well. I probably would have stayed in there if I was well but I began to think I couldn't cope with it anymore.

My mum found me unconscious in the bedroom, called an ambulance and I went into hospital. My relationship with my family was never really that good. My dad hit me a lot when I was young and I always felt very frightened of him. My mum's relationship with him was, well, she was quite subservient but she was supportive to us and did a lot for us as children. It was just my dad that was very aggressive and used to hit my mum and hit me. I was the oldest. I was actually quite scared of him even when I was in the Navy. I suppose that had a bit to do with my illness.

Because I was in the forces and they've got their own medical services, they took me to see a Navy doctor where I was based. I remember I spoke for hours about what was in my head. I just went on and on about delusions that were going on. I spent months in the hospital there. I was highly dosed up. I remember not being able to get up because they made me feel so drowsy. You fight it in a way, the medication, and then you feel so lethargic. We used to have to sit in circles, in chairs all the same height. We'd just sit there in silence with some of the staff and no one would say anything. They'd just leave it in silence, until someone said something *(laughs)*. Mostly we'd just sit there in silence and there would be someone shaking you know, with their medication. I think the Naval way of doing it was a short, sharp sort of shock kind of thing. They used to give you huge doses of medication whereas I know in a general hospital you'd have as little as possible. After nine months they discharged me from the hospital and the Navy.

I remember feeling distanced from everybody and having the feeling that I was going to have to cope with this for a long time. It's understandable why you feel depressed really. You know you've been happy, had a good life and interacted with people, had a good job and things are looking good in your career. And then suddenly you know its not there anymore. There's nothing to fill the day with.

I found it hard to get a job. I was still quite young and wanted to go back to work. After a year and a half I worked for the car parks being a car park attendant on sort of light duties. They liked me there and so they promoted me to a car park inspector, which isn't the best of jobs *(laughs)*. But I came off medication altogether when I was doing that. I was doing so much exercise during the day. Walking round the car parks, checking for tickets, to see if they'd got tickets, if they hadn't then maybe they'd gone for change and if they were not back within ten minutes, perhaps you'd give them a ticket. But I tried not to have too many confrontations. I think fitness has got a lot to do with mental health and making you feel better. I was there for a year and a half and didn't take any medication. Then I got a job in BT, as an engineer. I got really stressed doing that and went back onto medication. I was doing different jobs, difficult jobs. There were a number of jobs to do in a day, it was quite technical and there was a lot to learn.

I had one friend though, we'd been to school together. We played chess together and had both worked in the Navy and in BT. So we'd got kind of a friendship that had gone on all the way through which was really good. One evening we were in a restaurant and there were six girls and it was one of their birthdays and my friend who I was with knew one of the girls. So we sat next to them and that was how I met my wife, my future wife. She was one of the six. At the start she didn't understand about my illness really and we did separate after a few months. But I won her heart really. I sort of said I had a mental health problem right from the start. And her sister and family thought that I wasn't suitable. But they were quite friendly to me and they always have been and my wife's been quite supportive really.

I found it very difficult when our daughter was first born. I found it hard being a parent. It was stressful and it coincided with my wife's brother dying. It's quite hard to look after a baby. You're getting up early and you're working and you're finding work stressful. In a one bedroomed flat you feel quite claustrophobic and closed in *(pauses)*. Eventually I had another breakdown and went back into hospital. They accepted me back at work afterwards and I sort of got over it. But except for that time working in the car parks, I've been ill since '84 really. Until today. I'm still on medication now *(pauses)*.

I worked for BT for ten years and then I became ill again. I separated from my wife and daughter for a year and a half. I just couldn't cope; I felt claustrophobic. In only two rooms. The stress of work. All the negative feelings. Wanting to move but not being able to. More and more pressure at work, being asked to do more and more things. Getting up early, driving long distances, getting home and caring for a young child. My wife didn't like me talking about it because it got her down. I had problems with the mortgage. I was on a second mortgage to try and cope. In three years, I owed £17,000. I was supposed to pay up and I didn't have it.

When I was first ill, I didn't realise the signs but this time I went to see the BT doctor. He came to the conclusion that the stress of work was too much for me. I was retired. I was medically retired from the Navy as well. Medically retired twice!

I got gradually more and more confident when I left BT. That's 4 years ago now. I see a Community Psychiatric

Nurse every month. I suppose I'm quite a positive person really. I like a nice sort of positive view. The major problem I had was with the flat. So I saw an advocate who helped me buy a house, a two bed roomed house. My wife and daughter moved back in when I got the house. That was after a year and a half of being on my own. You think it's good being on your own. You've got freedom and that but I felt I needed company really and I felt that was better for me. I was having lots of microwave meals. I didn't have much enthusiasm when I was on my own *(pauses)*. I didn't like being on my own. Not being able to talk to anyone. A lot of people who have mental health problems are single, you know, living on their own and I looked round and I didn't want to do that. I don't want to do that. But a relationship, it's hard, you have to work at it, don't you?

A psychiatrist recommended I used a day service and it's working quite well really. I've been told that I do too much because I go to lots of meetings *(laughs)*. Local implementation team meetings with heads of Social Services and Health and other people and strategy meetings and mapping meetings. Lots of them. I've got a folder here of different work that I'm doing. But I get quite involved, you see. I do sport with a young people's place. They've all got a dual diagnosis. Some of them are into drugs as well as having mental health problems. We play football at the local sports centre and that's good. Also, I'm part a Forum that we set up to do User Focused Service Monitoring where we go round and interview other service users. Also I do other interviews. Interviews for employing staff. I've been trained how to do it.

Basically I feel like I'm working and that I'm giving a bit back. Sometimes I do feel a bit down about the future. A few people feel, you know, have the attitude 'why aren't you working?' towards me. Sometimes I feel a pressure that I should be working and maybe I might feel more complete or something, better in my mind if I was working. That's one thing that's stuck in my mind about the future but my CPN says fill out this form and you can be on this benefit for a while. So I get a little bit of money and that keeps me going. I'm not going to be rich or anything but it keeps me going. Stress can bring on the illness, bring on an episode. So the less stress I have the less I'm burdening society really.

My wife and I are very good parents. Our daughter has lots of friends at school. I have time to give a lot of help to my daughter which is good. Some parents are away from their children and can't give them much support. At the moment I'm quite happy really. Yeah, I've had a holiday in Majorca recently. First one for quite a few years. The first one my daughter's ever had. Well we've been to holiday camps before, you know like Haven holidays in Britain. But this was the first time abroad. It was fantastic. Big hole in the pocket, but fantastic.

Linda

Startlingly open and with a real need to talk about her experiences; both her arms were bandaged from where she had cut herself. When I met her, Linda was living in Sheltered Accommodation. After giving this interview Linda was admitted back into an acute psychiatric ward, at a hospital that has since closed down. She did not return to her previous accommodation and it has proved impossible to keep in touch with her.

I was born in Reading. At the age of three I watched my twin brother get run over by a car. He died instantly. It goes from that to now, to my older brother abusing me. I was raped three weeks ago by my brother. The in-between bits I have been trying to come to terms with it all, you know. The police were involved three weeks ago and also when I was a child. When I was about thirteen I spoke to Childline and they phoned my head of year or whatever they are called. She took me to one side and I explained it all to her. Five minutes later there was police there and social workers and stuff like that. You know so …(*long pause*)

My mum just tried to ignore me for the first six years after my brother died. She couldn't deal with the fact that I was still there and my twin wasn't. She never showed any love or care towards me. She didn't want nothing to do with me. She used to palm me off to the neighbours so they could look after me. She would leave my brother to look after

77

me when he was home and that's when it started. When it happened with him, do you know what I mean? When I was about thirteen he'd lock me in the bathroom after abusing me. He would tie something to my hand and then tie it to the banister so I couldn't get out of the room. Out of pure desperation I started cutting myself and that has gone on for years and years. Cutting and burning and stuff like that was like my way of coping with the situation. Because I was locked in the bathroom and couldn't get out and I figured the only way to cope with that was to cut myself. I started to self-harm when I was thirteen and I'm now twenty-eight, you know, so it's a long time.

I thought that by cutting myself I was getting rid of the dirt that was inside me. Seeing the dirt made me relax. I felt so filthy inside. I used to scrub myself probably ten times a day or whatever just to get rid of it. If I couldn't do that I'd cut myself you know or burn myself. There's not a lot more I can say about it really. It makes me feel a lot better if I cut myself because I still feel the past. I still feel trapped in the past. But now I'm trying to survive on the outside. I've been out of hospital for eighteen months now and I can say I'm a survivor of the mental health system.

I spent two years in a locked clinic. I couldn't cope so I set fire to my flat but it was horrible being in the locked clinic. I got attacked so many times, I lost count you know. I've been assaulted four times in hospital care. The first time I was sexually assaulted by another patient. The second time I was raped by another patient. The third time some patient chucked a cup of tea on my head, which is why I've got a scar on my head now. The fourth time was just recently while I was here; someone slammed a door into me and I got bruised all the way down. It's like the system don't really care. They put you in places like that and basically if another patient attacks, you can't do nothing about it. Because they say he's mentally ill he doesn't know what he's doing.   It really frustrates me you know. I think at the end of the day everyone knows what they are doing whether they are mentally ill or not. To a certain degree they actually know what they're doing, you know.

The place I was in was forensic. It was difficult. You're only allowed out twice a day for fifteen minutes a time. You have to eat at certain times and it's very institutionalised. I was just very mixed up; I didn't know what I was doing. I've got personality disorder and when I get ill, I get ill so there not a lot I can do about it. If someone gets ill with schizophrenia you can tell. If some one gets ill with personality disorder no one knows. You can't tell because that person is so complex. No one can even tell what illness it is. You know and if they can't find an illness they just say it's personality disorder. And that label got such a stigmatisation. I can't go to any support groups around here because I'm victimised because of the name. I wanted to go to one day centre but was told I couldn't because I had personality disorder. I wanted to go to another and they said I couldn't because I've got a forensic history. You know it's like you're victimised for having a personality disorder. Some people with personality disorder can carry on and lead a normal life. I say normal, there'd still be a lot of cutting and burning and a bit of uncontrollable behaviour.

When I get ill I start getting voices, I get stressed out. It's normally stress that brings it on… (long pause) and I either cut myself or burn myself. And I don't do it superficially either do you know what I mean? It's like this you know (shows bandaged arm).

I don't know why people have got this thing about personality disorders. It's just the way the system is at the moment …(long pause). I mean there is so much publicity at the moment about people with personality disorders anyhow. It's quite frustrating at times because I want to do something outside of the house and I can't because I'm stuck in here twenty-four hours a day. After a while that can really get to you. The last six weeks I've been self-harming quite a bit because I've got nothing to do and people have been stressing me out and stuff like that. Some times I self-harm out of boredom but not all the time… *(pauses)*

We get on really well me and my dad, we always have done. Mum's alright as well. I like my mum and dad, they're alright. I feel angry with them sometimes because they won't accept what my brother's done. They say, 'oh no my son couldn't have done that' and all the rest of it. They think I've gone against the family. I feel pretty powerless with my brother. I can't say leave me alone or whatever. He's got such a power over me. Like say I go home for the weekend, it's like a nightmare the whole time I'm at home. Last time I went home, about three weeks ago, I got raped and I got bruises all over me and stuff like that. My mum and dad had gone out of the house. It was the day of my uncle's funeral.... and I got home and he was there .... (*starts to cry*). Anyway, I don't want to go into it but yeah. I went to the police about it though and I'm not sure how that's going to turn out yet.

Why do I go back to my mum and dad's? Because I love my mum and dad and I want to see them. If it means having to see him then that's the way it's gotta be. Both Mum and Dad are disabled now you see and I can't really leave them all week. I have to go home on a Friday and come back on a Monday just to look after them over the weekend. But it makes life extremely hard having to go back home and look after them the whole time. It's like I'll be cooking the dinner, doing the washing up and doing this and doing that, do you know what I mean?

I go out quite a bit like around town and stuff like that during the week. You know so it's quite good. Also, I've got eight chaffinches in my room so I'm always looking after them. Going down the shop to get stuff for them. They're quite good, the only thing is they get me up at half three in the morning. Starting a fight, the male and the female. Typical male female relationship really. They make a noise, a really squeaky noise. And when I turn the light off at night they both decide to go mad with their wings, flying around the cage. They'll be like that till about one in the morning and I'm like 'go to sleep *please*'… *(pauses)*. And I've got fish too. The other day I found one in the filter and it was dead. I got it out of the water and I waved it above the tank and said to the other fish "see that" I said " that's what happens to you when you fly into the filter". *(laughs)* Yeah, I spend a lot of my time looking after the animals I've got in my room. Like cleaning them out and stuff like that, you know. I want to get a rabbit but they won't let me have a rabbit here because we're too near the main road *(laughs)*. Plus there is nowhere to put a hutch that is out of the way.

I've got a voluntary job on a Tuesday. It's with Action for Children. It's for children who have witnessed their parents being raped or murdered, brothers being killed and stuff like that you know. I do that from one till five every Tuesday, so that's quite good. I just went round there and said have you got a job going and they said "yeah " and so I started *(laughs)*. I just pack in the back room. I get the clothes folded, tag 'em, price 'em and put 'em out on the shelves. Sort through all the stuff that people have sent in, you know it's quite good. I quite enjoy that.

Well when I think about the future... I forgot to tell you some stuff actually. I've got a son as well which I forgot to mention. He'll be twelve in February. He lives in care in Devon. He's doing really well for himself. He's got Asperger's Syndrome so that causes him to be in his own world all the time and a lot of this... a lot of repetitive talk. But he's doing reasonably OK (sighs). He likes it where he is. He writes to me and I write to him. It's pretty good.

I haven't seen him for about five years now. I care about him but I was living in hospital and they didn't think it was a good idea for me to see him whilst I was there, so in the end we just drifted apart. But we still write to each other. The foster mother writes to me every two weeks to let me know how he's doing and she sends me photos of him and stuff like that, that's pretty good. I didn't even know who the father was until he was born... *(laughs)*. It was a choice of three so yeah.... The easy bit about it was his dad was Indian and there was also two white blokes. So when he was born I knew. This dark baby came out. And I thought 'Aha, I know who the father is now.' (laughs) Yeah really weird. His dad doesn't even know he exists. He left the country as soon as he found out I was pregnant because I'd only just turned sixteen at the time. I was what you call 'jail bait' - you remember that saying? (laughs) Yeah so... I put him in care when he was three. I couldn't cope with him, I was in and out of hospital all the time. I didn't think it was very fair on him to have to put up with that. So I put him in care for his own sake, you know really. Well to be a normal child. Yeah he seems pretty normal. He's just got problems you know. Same sort of problems like 'Why did my mum put me in care?' and 'Why can't I see my family?' and stuff like that.... Normal questions that an eleven year old would say. Maybe when he gets a bit older he'll understand a bit more.

At the moment he's very confused, he doesn't really understand why he was put into care. All I've ever told him is what I say in the letters. Right from when he was five I used to write to him and say 'mummy's got a poorly head. That's why she's in hospital.' I couldn't say something like 'mummy's got a personality disorder' because he wouldn't have had a clue what I was on about, do you know what I mean? So I put it in the simplest terms and its like he understands that. So he's pretty good about that... (pauses)

I'm with a new bloke now. I've been going out with him for the last year. We are planning to get a flat together when we leave here, maybe have some children, I don't know. We haven't decided yet. We have got a future planned but the main thing is getting out of here. I'm not being funny but when you're well you're well and if you're around people who are unwell, it can make you unwell again. I don't know if I could handle it if I got unwell again. So it's best to get out of here while I still can *(laughs)*. Do you know what I mean?... *(pauses)* I'm optimistic about the future but you know how it is...If it comes it comes. I take each day as it comes, I don't bother planning like months ahead. I just take each day as it comes. You know that's like, my way of coping. I take it each day as it comes because I find if I plan too far ahead it doesn't work and then I get quite distressed about it, you know. So I have to think day to day, it's just a lot better for me... *(pauses)*.

My boyfriend lives just there. Right next door virtually. Handy! We usually go to each other's rooms, listen to music. We've both got those fibre optic lights and they're quite cool. I'd like candles but we can't have them because of the fire alarms here.

It was in hospital that I found out that there was people a lot iller than what I was. That made things quite difficult really. You'd wake up in the morning and think: 'Am I going to get hit today?', 'Am I going to get punched today?', 'Is someone going to beat me up?'... (pause). In the end you just give up. Sometimes in the end there's no point in defending yourself. I mean I spent most of the time under twenty-four hour observation, when I was in the locked clinic. They saw self-harm as a life threatening thing when it wasn't. You know, it's the same as if you broke your arm really. If you broke your arm, you don't like not get it treated. You go to hospital and you get it sorted. Self-harm's the same thing really. If you cut yourself, you go and get it sorted. When it's superficial and you're put on twenty-four obs for just scratching yourself you know, it's all wrong. They don't understand the difference between suicidal people and people just cutting themselves. They presume that because you cut yourself you are suicidal. Yeah, that's why they put you in locked wards, someone watching you the whole time. Yeah, the system's all wrong. They've got no understanding of self-harm really. I mean at the end of the day it doesn't matter how many jobs you go to, how many courses you do, you still won't know what its like to be a self harmer. It's a lack of understanding in the mental health system. You know to the point where when I was in the locked clinic I got the policy changed on self-harm. You know so that people wouldn't get moved out of their rooms or get their rooms stripped. Stuff like that or have their clothes taken away and being put in strips, like the old Victorian times in a hospital.

I felt suicidal loads of times. I took loads of overdoses but it never worked. I started off taking things like paracetemol when I was in school. I took a hundred paracetemol in one day. That was like taking two every ten minutes all through the day. You don't feel the difference but in the end you pass out. When I passed out I got rushed to hospital and that's when they found out I'd took the overdose. Lucky they managed to sort me out otherwise I wouldn't be here now.

It had just come out about my brother and I was getting a lot of grief at home and that's why I took the overdose. I thought well, no-one loves me, no one wants me sort of thing, I might as well kill myself. That's why I tried to kill myself at thirteen. I've been in and out of psychiatric units since then. I've been out eighteen months now. That's cool, isn't it?

There wasn't a point where I decided to change, it happened on its own accord *(laughs)*. Just thinking about the future is the only thing that keeps me well. Like I said I go from day to day but I do look towards the future as well. Sometimes I set goals for the future and if I achieve them I give myself a pat on the back, do you know what I mean?. My psychologist has helped me quite a bit and that's quite nice. Her name's Patsy. She talked about my problems and tried to get to the root of things. I used to have to do exams and tests and things like that. To find out what was really wrong with me. I had to do silly things like building blocks and things like that to find out if I had learning difficulties, which I knew I didn't but they were convinced I did. So I did the tests and of course then they said 'no she hasn't got learning difficulties'. I went 'ha'. *(laughs)* Yeah, you know they were trying to give me something I ain't got. I'd know if I'd had learning difficulties.

When I was in hospital I learnt about different coping mechanisms: thought stopping, ways of dealing with anger and stuff like that. I did little groups and I suppose they were quite helpful really. Some of them seemed a bit stupid at times but they did help. It seemed a bit unrealistic really. Like they'd give you a scenario, you had three people in your group and you all had to play a part, like one had to play the father, one the son and one the daughter. The father had just crashed his car and the son and daughter were giving advice but they didn't know how to. We all had to play different parts. I suppose it was quite good.

The staff here have been pretty supportive. Mum and Dad's been alright too and that's all I need really. I need support as well as a home. A wish for the future is having a husband and children. And having a home would be like …. It'd be good. One day it'll happen.

Peter

Pete is fifty-two years old and has been coping with depression and anxiety for over twenty years. He describes himself as 'stuttering and shy' and of low self-esteem. When I met him he was friendly and open in talking about his experiences. He has a degree in Housing Studies and is currently undertaking voluntary work for several organisations.

I do suffer from paranoia but I think to a certain extent that it's justified. I think some mental health workers, 'depend' on certain members - or 'patients', or 'clients' or whatever they call people who use their services. They perhaps can't accept that these people are moving on, or moving up or moving out. Or just don't need them anymore. I was talking about this very thing with a schizophrenic friend yesterday evening. The topic came up and *(laughs)*...we agree.

He said, 'there's some who can't believe you can get to and from the city centre by yourself.' Now, these are sweeping libellous generalisations but over the past five years, despite having had this type of conversation with one of them, some mental health workers still treat me very much as a patient. I went to an allotment fete in August. Great day. I met a worker from a drop-in centre that I used to go to. When I saw her, the first thing she does is tell me where their stall is, and I thought, I don't want to know where it is. I've not been to the centre for months. I've *worked* for them, doing some driving. It really annoyed me. So that's one aspect of my particular situation.

I started at working at Oxfam on the road to decent paid work. Stuffing envelopes in the packing area. Some staff there think of me as someone who works in the packing department - that particular department is for disabled people – despite the fact I've done quite responsible clerical jobs in other departments. I think they're a bit cliquish anyway up there. Another libel I suppose.*(laughs)* I only spend one and a half hours there per week now. In fact it's down to every two weeks. Two weeks in a month. It's because of illness that I've cut it down. In fact, I've been encouraged to do more, which I've been nervous about taking on.

I presume my colleagues must socialise with each other. With all the centres and office staff that there are. People who work in mental health are not allowed to meet members outside of their work. Some are even stricter. None of the workers who have contracts are allowed to have a sexual relationship with the members. Which is because of the law and exploitation. I get…I mean, I can see some sense in that.

To put it in a wider context though, if it's part of the constitution, or culture, or ethos of mental health organisations to encourage users/members to move on, including working for them, or working on the mental health scene, then the social aspect is a problem. You feel you aren't being accepted as a colleague, that you're still regarded as a member of a drop-in centre. The more one is – I'll use quotes - 'rejected' by them, the more one is kept in the circles of one's – quote - 'loony' friends. I've nothing against loony friends but you're... *(pauses)*. I just don't want to be on the scene anymore. I will choose who I want as friends whether, however they're defined.

Oxford's not the friendliest place anyway so trying to break out of that scene, those circles, well it's still galling in a way. When all you've got after five years is the friends you had before you started to do other work, most of whom you've met on the mental health scene, as members and users. And it's a big problem. I mean mainly because Oxford is so unfriendly, it's hard to make friends, especially not working full-time anywhere. So I think that's a problem, a general problem for any organisation wanting to use our expertise or experience in being a service user. There still seems to be a bit of apartheid. You know, if I were to move to a different city, I'd try not to be a member of a mental health drop-in centre. So that it would be a clean sheet as it were, but here, in Oxford, well it's impossible.

I wouldn't say I'm OK now though. That's the other side of the coin. I mean we are told that it is not them and us. That people are not completely ill or completely well, it's not black or white and so it's bound to be somewhere in between. However you define yourself. Whichever door you walk through. I mean whether you walk through the patients' door or the doctors' door. Well I have anxiety and depression. And some physical problems.

I started work again – that's a sign of getting better for me. Of recovering. I started work about ten years ago. Stuffing envelopes for half a day. Mainly through invitation by different employers, I expanded that to about sixteen hours a week or more. Of course, if that were found out by the DSS I wouldn't qualify for incapacity benefit and that is another aspect of this sort of journey. I suppose it's a sign of progress anyway. The peak of work achievements was about a year ago but unfortunately I got made redundant from the second best job that I had. Well, it was all tailing off anyway and in fact, I walked out once I realised, well, what was happening.

Work can be great. It can be great company, give you the feeling that you're doing something useful, with the responsibility and the sense of achievement. I suppose it's tangible in what I do: posters, flyers, newsletters, being responsible for people when I'm driving. Also I know it's good in the longer term to build confidence; experience; a CV. I was a manager for five years. I'd like to get back to the sort of person I was then. Sometimes the stuff I do now can be a bit boring at times and I do end up thinking then 'what am I doing this for?' When I *can* do this or that and I *used* to do the other *(pauses)*...

One of the cleaners said, about what was a voluntary job: 'What couldn't they afford you, Pete?' *(laughs)* Which is quite funny but quite cruel as well. I mean you've got to be pretty bad to be made redundant from a voluntary job. They didn't even pay my expenses. I think it was to do with personalities. Different people moved into the office in which I worked. Including a new boss. But that's life I suppose. It helps a great deal though to go to work. I must confess that I find it hard to entertain myself as it were. I live on my own in a bedsit in an area that's unfriendly and I've not made any friends there. Well I've made one friend in the house and that can make all the difference but he works full-time. I don't want to bother him too much. So I spread my work over four days. Friday, is my free day. I deliberately set it up like that in order to be working when the drop-in centre is open, 'uh so I wasn't tempted to go back there.

I don't want to go to the drop-in centre on principle. I realise I've got to make it, well perhaps not on my own but without people who are paid to help me. Paid to be nice. Paid to listen. So called 'befriending', when I know that they're not allowed to meet me outside of their work. That's not friendship at all, that's part of a job. It's not real life. It's not what the world is like. You've got to make it on your own in that sense. So those are the reasons... A friendly acquaintance of mine in a similar relationship with the drop-in centre said a few years ago, after he'd stopped going, that the place was great at getting you to a certain level and then keeping you there. So it's very interesting. I still don't think I've told any of the people that work there that. I'd like to.

What eventually clinched it was this job that I eventually got made redundant from. There was a new company that took over which meant computerisation and all that sort of stuff. They said they would train me on the computer to do the job I was doing. I thought well, if they've got that much faith in me, then that's great, I should have some faith in them. It felt good. Around the same time I can remember sitting at the drop-in in the afternoon, having had a so-called 'chat', with a worker. It seemed that we were allowed around one 'chat' a day, which I suppose is fair enough. I was sitting there looking around and thinking 'what have I got in common with most members here, except problems? And being ill.' Very little positive or neutral, or indifferent. In other words, 'why am I here?' It was useful to talk with a worker. Or literally chat with a worker. Workers rather. Other than that, I had to ask myself the question 'why am I here?' Those two things came along around about the same time. That was when I re-jigged my week so that I wouldn't be tempted to go back there again.

I think I've come to realise that what's useful, what some of us need (people in recovery or perhaps, sadly, getting worse and going downhill) is a very low level of support. Something that's available if you need it but you probably won't. I mean I've been to the Samaritans a few times in the past five years. As a deliberate alternative to going to a drop in centre because I didn't want to go back to that. So in sort of, broader, general terms there's a need for that, for a lower level of support.

This is the first time I've thought about it like that. I mean the encouragement, the empowerment, is there from certain individuals. I've benefited enormously from one of them and I thank them still. I feel I need encouragement in 'developing'. Yes, I mean I'm happy here and in other forums to describe myself as ill, mentally ill but I know there's more I could do and can do, did do.

How do I define myself? It depends who's asking? How I feel at the time. I'm certainly a lot more than a mentally ill person, a 'patient'. Because as I've said I'm a driver now and it's the most responsible job I've ever done. I drive people, not parcels. I'm also a DTP operator. An Editor of a newsletter. Unattached...childless. Poor. A bit intellectual, a bit academic but can also be quite practical. I was mending something the other week...so yeah I suppose I can be quite practical. That's good.

I've travelled a lot and I recently went to Paris. The trip was a prize. I found it very nerve-wracking but I'm so glad I did it. I had all sorts of fears including practical ones, because of physical problems. The best part of it was that there wasn't a mental worker in sight. Or if there was, they weren't in that role. I was a bit panicky and clingy the first morning, and asked two people if I could go with them into town because the hotel was in the suburbs. You had to catch a bus and then a train. I have an obvious stutter and I felt very self-conscious about it so I asked to accompany them. As I was saying earlier, I didn't need developing as such but encouragement to develop. Anyway I latched on to these two to help me catch the bus and then change and catch the train. I got off at Notre Dame as they suggested and they carried on. After that I did do it all by myself largely... *(pauses)* which in a way is pathetic, given that I've travelled by myself across the States. And I've hitched to Greece. But things like that were all before I was ill. Since I've been ill...well I did, hitch to Amsterdam but I didn't feel as nervous doing that. I don't know why but going to Paris felt like the biggest achievement of this sort.

I'd say I fell ill nineteen years ago when I was travelling in Ireland. I'd been going through some funny states at home where I was in my last year at Oxford poly doing a postgraduate certificate. I was having counselling every week there. I was in some pretty bad states, it was quite frightening at times.

I'd done my ankle in, in England, but I'd sort of persevered and that made it worse. I had to see a quack in Dublin because I was literally limping. We ended up changing our plans from hitching to going by train. I suppose I felt like I was a burden to the people I was with. I decided to stay in my tent while they went out. I was having funny ideas while I was in there. Of fire and flames and being burnt, in the tent. It was pretty nasty. Shortly afterwards they went off again and did something else by themselves.

I may have been hallucinating. I can't really recall. I've not really talked about it in such detail before. But again the physical symptoms and things were there and I definitely couldn't cope. Especially because of this bloody ankle, my Achilles heel. I would call it a near breakdown that I was going through or heading for.

I was due to meet them at the station to travel, say Westwards or Southwards. So I decided to travel Eastwards by myself and just go, just sort of withdraw from it all. It brought things to a head. Certainly I was suffering from anxiety or over anxiety. Part of it, although I may not have realised it then, was being away from home and safety. If you are hitching or even just travelling away from home, you're poor and you're camping. That's all a lot of effort. Having to cook for yourself and things.

I'd been to the States and Mexico in 1980…The States was not half as dangerous then as it's reputation. It was a place that I'd wanted to go to since 1969, on hearing a song called 'In America' by Simon and Garfunkel. On the album, 'Bookends.' So that was a great ambition finally achieved and it was a holiday of a lifetime. It was travelling really, not a holiday. Trying to find work. I'd read 'On The Road' by Jack Kerouac twice. I probably had more money in the States than in Ireland as well. You don't have to make choices between making your foot worse or catching a bus. You'd just catch the bus.

In Ireland I'd suffered physical injury. Which literally makes you more vulnerable. And pain. Physical pain. Also I'm wondering about these two friends. Of course they were good in that they'd changed their plans and it involved spending more money, going by train rather than hitching.

But to be honest I felt a bit let down by them. I was actually jealous of them going off by themselves while I was having a rest day…. I did have a very bad irritable colon at the time. I was going to the toilet about 7 or 8 times a day. Which again when you're camping causes practical problems. Bowel breaks. You feel as if you're drained, weak; not physically well.

I have what my acupuncturist calls attacks which include feeling very sleepy in the afternoon. I'd had them on and off for five years or so but they were getting more frequent then. So I was even less with it in the afternoons.

I do have plans for the future. It tends to be the day to day, day by day sort of thing but I would like to live with someone eventually. I think I'm too old for children now. I would like to end up with average income, that would be fantastic. An average graduate income. To get a decent job. I'd like to be out of debt. These aren't plans so much as wishes, I suppose. But 'er *(pauses)*…a decent home, however I interpret that. In general though my view of things is that it's a bit pointless aiming for perfection in life because that life is just different levels of imperfection.

If I could perhaps think a little more on a shallow level and in the short term, it might perhaps be better than thinking deeply and in the long term as I do. I do too much of that really. I'd like to survive at Christmas. *(laughs)* That's a plan.

When I was in Paris at Le Place de la Bastille, I was trying to pluck up courage to ask for a cup of coffee in a café. I got really annoyed at myself and was determined that I would not let fear rule my life and that I would not live regretful of things I hadn't done. I had to do sort of anxiety management thinking. Say to myself 'Oh alright then Pete, you're nervous. So be it. You still want do that thing. You won't have the opportunity after a day or two. There's no-one here to help you.'

I can remember walking around the outside of the roundabout in front of the café, and thinking 'come on Pete, for God's sake. Jesus Christ. What does it matter if you fuck up, at least you can get a cup of coffee. What's the big deal?' *(laughs)* So...and I did it and it was great. It was a very valuable experience.

Have I mentioned my acupuncturist? I've been having acupuncture for nineteen years. I think that's saved my life on more than one occasion. I swear by it. It's about energy flow. Called Chi energy. Which is the same Chi as in T'ai Chi. Shiatsu, for example, is pressure on acupuncture points. It changes the energy flow of a particular organ or emotion. It's all a bit airy fairy and 'er... intangible but it's worked for umpteen thousand years.

With complimentary medicine, it's a partnership you see. You can't just take pills or get an operation and get better. You've got to work at it yourself *(laughs)*. So I would emphasise that aspect of mental health as well. I know that I could do more. In the end I think it's down to us. For all the chats with the workers. Or cups of tea. Or cheap meals. Or advice. Or courses. In the end it's down to the individual to make... well, at that stage it might not even be an effort.

Anne

I met Anne on a truly awful day weather wise. We sat in a dark room above the day centre she attended while she told me her story. Throughout our talk the rain was unremitting, slashing against the windows. It seemed apt somehow; Anne, a thin, frail woman has suffered from depression for many years. Anne lives alone and has two grown-up children.

My mother used to tie me in the chair when I was a child because I would never sit still. She used to say to my sister, "She will sit still". My sister was four years older and would ridicule me, you know. She was a mother who was too possessive over her children. I was very well looked after, put it that way, and she took me to the doctors numerous times when I was a child. Of course, in those days you had to pay but money was irrelevant. Often I wouldn't eat. I was dreadful for eating, and the doctor advised her to take me to the chemist and buy numerous things. Some of it was horrible and she used to make me take it.

We were a middle class family. We weren't poor and we weren't rich. My father was lovely and I suppose my mother was too really. My life was a ritual though. You get up, you have your breakfast, you go to school, come home, midday meal on the table. Go back to school, come home and then have tea at four o'clock, then it would be into your bedrooms or another room in the house. Father would come home and we weren't allowed to speak to him till he'd had his evening meal and then it was bath and bed. Sitting up with a book. Even in the summer holidays. It was all a ritual. But they were very good, you know.

I must have been born restless though. I can remember I hadn't been married long. We had a rented flat because at the time we had to save up money to buy a place of our own. And I hadn't been married for more than two or three months when I ran out of the flat thinking, 'I've got to get away, I've got to get away'. I went to the pictures on my own. I sat in there for about an hour and then I came back and I can remember my husband crying, saying things like "perhaps you shouldn't have married me. Perhaps this isn't good enough for you". Silly things, you know. I think all my life I've always been thinking and feeling that - that I've got to get out. That I couldn't sit still.

I've been diagnosed with depression for about thirty years. My son was ten when I was first put on medication. I was very low. He came home from school one day and I said "I've taken a whole bottle of tablets". He was very good. He got on the phone and called the police and they sent an ambulance along. It was following that that I first went into a mental hospital. In London. It was a horrible institution, a very old Victorian building. They put me in there. I'll always remember it, it was so old and horrible. The nurses wore white coats and that'll always stay in my mind. One of them gave us brooms and told us to sweep the floor. We had a bed with a small wardrobe thing attached to it. When we'd finished sweeping, she said 'polish it' and I thought, 'this is just dreadful'.

It's gone away for spells, the depression, but it's always come back. I've just been to see my psychiatrist today in fact, Dr Stevens - I relate to him you know. I get good days and I get bad days. It's dreadful really, very wearing. An awful thing. I do drive because I live on my own since I've lost my husband. I tend to drive down the coast road and sit staring at the sea for hours and hours. As I was saying I've always had this feeling that I've got to get out of the house and go somewhere away, as if I'm trying to find something that's not there.

I've been in so many hospitals in London, because I came from London before we moved down here. One hospital I went to, in Harrow: I can remember going into the hospital, into that old Victorian hospital and I said to the psychiatrist there,

'I loathe coming into your building'.

He said 'Why?' and I said, 'It's that grotty, old grey entrance'.

I used to think 'Oh God have I got to go through there?' A couple of months after that, I'd had to go back again and see him and they were painting it.

I said to him 'That's lovely isn't it'.

And he said 'We do listen to the patients you know'. I'll always remember that.

I was nineteen when I met my husband. His sister and I went to a dance. It was in a Catholic church hall. We were friends, my sister in-law and I and she didn't like going home at night on her own. That night she said, 'My brother, Michael, is coming to meet me. To take me home. He doesn't like me going home on my own.' So he came to pick her up and it ended up with us seeing Jayne home first and then him taking me back *(laughs)*. I had a wonderful husband, he always wanted to please me. He would do anything for me. I grieve for him tremendously.

My husband and his sister were very close and they were so much alike. They had to do what they wanted to do, you know. I think sometimes he thought I couldn't handle things. He had to be the one that had to handle everything. Even money and things like that, he did everything. He did all the banking. He did everything that had to be done. But he was very good. He'd say to me "If you want any money, just go to the bank". I had a card. He'd say go and get yourself some money, if you want to buy clothes or do some shopping. He never quibbled over money. Which was wonderful really.

But depression is like you're down in a black hole and you can't get out. People don't understand what it's like until they've been through it. My husband was very good though. He was a sort of ad-lib type of person and he'd come into a room and if there was a crowd of people, after a few minutes he'd come out with something and he'd have them all laughing. Numerous people over the years have said he should have been a comedian. On the stage you know, because he was, well, he wasn't a forceful man, and he wouldn't push himself to anybody, but he was just that type of person. He had charisma. I think he understood what I'd been through all those years. He was the only person that really did, I think, you know. He used to make a joke of it. He used to say to my daughter "Oh, mum's gone again" and roll his eyes. And I used to say "Oh shut up'. I haven't been able to explain it to anyone else though, how you get to the stage when you get angry with yourself. You get angry and just think 'why, why?'

I don't think even they understand it, the psychiatrists I mean, what depression is. It lasts for such a long time. You're down there and it can go on and on. You can't sleep at night and it's like a spinning top going round and round. Everything, all the thoughts just going round and round all the time.

I loved my children. I really did. I did everything for them. But I think, I don't even think they understood. I mean, when you think, my boy, only ten years of age and going in an ambulance with me to the hospital. Of course he didn't understand. And I worry. I think I hope my daughter hasn't got my genes. Or my son. I don't think I've seen anything there but you never know, do you? My daughter, I think, is more like her father. He could handle anything. She's wonderful really. She always aims to please people. She's got a lovely disposition, like her dad. She's got three boys, one of sixteen, one of eleven and one of seven. The way she handles them boys. When I see them all sitting on the settee, the three of them falling on her. And my son in-law. Four big lumps I say. I think it's lovely though.

My son's got two girls. One's nine and one's seven. I don't talk to my daughter in-law. It was some years ago now....about seven maybe. She came to my home and her other little girl was only about three then and she put a shoe to her mouth, and my daughter in law, she jumped up quickly and said 'if you don't take that shoe from your mouth I'm going to hit you'. I jumped up and said " Sharon, she hasn't done anything", and she ran out to the car crying and I ran upstairs. My son brought the eldest girl in his arms to say goodbye and I thought "Gosh, what have I done?" She did run out crying. So the following day it was her birthday, on the Saturday, and I bought a birthday card and I bought Marks + Spencer's vouchers for her birthday and went over to the house and didn't get any answer. My husband said 'What are you going to do?' and I said 'I don't know' and he said, 'Oh, just put it through the letter box'. And from that day my daughter in law hasn't spoken to me. So cruel.

I still see my son. My son came down the Saturday before last. He came down on Saturday and we went through the town and then we went along the beach with the girls and then we went out and had a meal.

I mustn't say anything really bad about my daughter in law because she's ....well, her house is so clean. The girls are really looked after so lovely. My son's looked after and truly, if you had a meal at her house you wouldn't get it any better if you'd been to one of these top chefs. She really is an excellent cook and you'd have beautiful meals. And, I don't know why, I don't know what it is, you know *(pauses)*.... I'm not the type of person to ever be vindictive about anybody. I would sooner help somebody than be that.

I have spoken to my son about it. Not brought it right to the fore, because it's a very delicate subject, isn't it? The little girl has said once "My mummy does really like you, but it's too late now", or something to that effect.

I get on wonderful with my son in-law though. He's my rock. He's done everything for my husband and I. He's a top ranking police officer but he's an honest police officer. He would never do anything that wasn't in the book, you know, and all his men like him because he's so straight. He's so likeable, he's marvellous. He'd do anything for me and my daughter. They've got their problems though. They've got a boy of sixteen and he walked out of school and he said, 'I don't like your school' to the headmaster. It's such a shame because he's got a marvellous brain. And he's just thrown it away. There were two in the whole school that got top marks for science and he was one of them and that's a hard subject isn't it? But he walked out of school, and anyway, they've had a lot of problems with him.

My depression never goes away. I get a lot of anxiety in my tummy. Some days I cook a meal and I can't eat it and I bin it. I've told the psychiatrist about it and he said 'I understand how you must feel at times'. And I do feel it. Sometimes, when I'm at the drop in centre with the group, I can't stop talking. I go on and on my head's saying 'you've got to stop, you've got to stop'. Mostly I'm not really a talker you know. I prefer to go along the coast on my own and sit for hours and hours.

Sometimes I'll just sit there and I think I'll call it a day[9]. I say to myself, 'shall I call it a day?' Then I cry. And I say to myself "You're not going to solve anything" and I suddenly think, 'What will my daughter think? What will my son think?' If I did it, they'd have to live with the fact that I've … you know. And then I think, well if you can say that you're not going too. Sometimes I've walked up the cliff road and I get thoughts of throwing myself off and things like that. The thoughts don't go away. They're there all the time.

Numerous times I have really hated myself and got a razor and cut my arms so bad. I get so angry with myself that I have kept on making them bleed. I think I've got to punish myself for being like it. I don't think that's something that'll ever go. I can't explain it. I think I've learned to live with it more now and have learnt more about it than what I have in the past. There were times then when I wasn't in control of myself and that made me keep going in and out of hospitals having treatment. In a way I think now I've come to terms with the fact that it'll always be there. I mean, I get some days when I'm very low and it will lift. It may lift at about 9 o'clock at night, just before going to bed and suddenly I'll think, I feel happy. I get my good days and I get my bad days. But except from going to the drop-in centre

---

[9] Anne talks here about the possibility of committing suicide.

and the support I get from that, I think I'm a loner. I keep myself to myself. I've never been a very good mixer.

I feel ashamed of myself. I talk to Dr Stevens and tell him about how I feel ashamed of myself. He says you haven't got anything to be ashamed of. He said he's had people who've had physical illnesses and depression and they've said that they would sooner have the physical illness than the depression.

I've taken the overdoses when I couldn't cope with the depression. When I've just wanted to finish myself you know. You get frightened; frightened of yourself really. You don't know what to do. You're mixed up. There were times when I thought my children and my husband would be better off without me and there were times when I just didn't have a thought for them. You don't you know. You're just gone. In a very deep depression, you're really gone. You don't remember anything afterwards. I was in hospital for three months once and I didn't think I was ever going to come out. It takes you over and it's as if you're not even in your own body. Your mind goes. You go. You don't even remember who your husband is. He came to visit me once and I kept thinking 'who is he?' I really did. I really was that bad. I've had ECT's[10] too. They can make your memory go.

---

[10] Electro Convulsive Therapy.

I can phone the CPNs[11] anytime. When I lost my husband, I phoned them at midnight. I had all my tablets, I had aspirin, I had nurofen, I had every tablet I could find in my drawer all together on the table and I was crying and I thought 'I'm going to take them'. I really wanted to talk to somebody, somebody who could help me and I phoned the CPN and they spoke to me for about an hour. In the end, I promised them I wouldn't take them and they said, 'Go to bed and you might feel a bit better tomorrow'. This was one o'clock in the morning. I just got in bed and there was a crash on my front door and it was two policemen. They'd sent two policemen. Two young lads at one o'clock in the morning. The tablets were still on the table. They half frightened me to death. They took every tablet because I really couldn't be sure that I wouldn't take the whole lot at some point during the night.

As I've said to Dr Stevens, I've even thought about going into Boots and getting two hundred aspirins or whatever you can get. I know they wouldn't serve me with a lot because they know that there's a reason. You don't usually buy that amount in one go. But then I thought about going to Superdrug and another chemist and buying some. That's the kind of things that go through your mind when

---

[11] Community Psychiatric Nurses.

you're depressed. It's a comforting thought to know it's there I suppose, if I need it.

In the past, I think that what used to upset me, and I have sat and cried over this, was that there didn't seem to be a reason for it. I've said to the psychiatrists 'can you find a reason for it?' They never could and that used to make me cry because I would get so angry and wish I had a reason. I wanted a reason why I'd got it. I used to think if you were disabled sitting in a chair and you couldn't move and things like that, and you were depressed, then you'd say well at least there's a reason, there's a cause. If you had something really wrong with you, then you've got a reason for feeling like it. I couldn't find any cause, that's what used to upset me. It still does. Why can't I find the answer to it. I've been to the library and got lots of books on depression and read and re-read them. Perhaps I go in too deep sometimes, over it all. You're trying to find an answer and what if there isn't one. I used to think to myself 'now you've got no problems'. And I haven't got any problems. I haven't got a husband that beat me up or anything like that. We weren't rich but we never had money problems. I would be happy if I could. I think if I knew why, then at least I could try and solve the problem and then I may not even get depression, I don't think, if I had a reason for it. If somebody could give me the answer, I'd be so happy. But there isn't an answer is there. That's, I think, the sad part about it.

I had a great grandmother who came from France and when I was a child she lived in London where I lived, with her son. She used to always be taken away. Of course now I think she must have been taken off into hospital but my mother never spoke about it. Mother never spoke about it. We did hear little bits though. They were always taking her away. Sometimes they say it's hereditary don't they? In the genes, you know. I often think … it's silly really. But you do look back at your family and think there could be something there, you know. That could have been the cause. It may not be at all. It may not have had anything to do with it.

Some days it lifts. Some days I can go high. Very high. The other doctor, Dr Bashir, wanted me to go on Lithium to stabilise my moods and I know it sounds silly, but one of the CPNs down there said I had to have blood tests for that and he'd never done a blood test before and there he was poking and prodding my arm to get this blood out and do you know, I went home and I suddenly thought 'I'm not taking this anymore.' And I refused to take it.

One day I was very high and I got in my car; I shouldn't have been driving really because I was that high. I went to Hythe, near Southampton. I parked my car and I got on a funny little train. It was a funny old-fashioned train you go on. Like a toy train. Then you get on the ferry and then you go over on the ferry. I went into Marks and I didn't half buy some clothes. I brought loads and loads of clothes and I was really high and I went in the Food Hall and I bought lots of things. I bought bottles of wine and everything and I was carrying these great big bags. I was getting onto the ferry and I was struggling. I knew I wasn't in control but something was telling me I had to do it. I could have flown round the world how I felt, you know. It's awful really. I couldn't carry them so this man had to help me. Then I got in the car and came home. I sat down and I made myself a cup of tea and I thought 'you silly woman, what are you doing all that for?' Well, I'd bought all those clothes and I wore them, but normally when I'm not high I wouldn't do things like that.

But I've got to the stage now where I've had so much medication. Over the years, every day, every hospital I've been in, it's like you're just giving up and taking the pills and you keep taking them. That's not the answer though, is it? I don't think so, no. When I look back over the years - thirty years I've had this - I've had so much medication. I suppose it has helped in a way, somewhere along the line, it must have, you know, when I've been well, but when I've gone down, I've really gone down and I wasn't even in control of myself. That's how depression takes people.

I've had psychologists, not here, but when I was in London. I used to see one every week. The last time I was in hospital was in London, you know. I used to see this lady psychologist and we used to talk and talk. I suppose it helped at the time, to off load your thoughts and how you feel and that, but it doesn't solve anything. No. It's just something like, I'd say it's just like a physical illness. You've got to live with it. If somebody's got something wrong with them, you know, like these people who've got physical illnesses, then sometimes it's not going to get better, it's always going to be there. Depression can be like that; a pain that doesn't go away. That's how I feel about it.

I get terrible butterflies sometimes, and I walk round the house. I walk up the stairs and walk down from one room to another. Silly things happen - I couldn't find a cardigan. It was a fairly new one - and I thought 'where is it?' The obsession over that cardigan made me ill. I pulled every cupboard out. I pulled the beds out, looked under the beds. I went everywhere in that house. I stripped my house completely to pieces. I never found that cardigan. It possessed me. I pulled the car inside out and I kept thinking 'have I been somewhere and taken my cardigan off and left it?' Then I thought 'have I left my car open sometime and somebody's taken it?' It was an obsession. I kept saying to myself 'Let go of it, let go of it. Go and buy yourself one. Go and buy yourself six'. It was worrying me so much and I don't know why because I've got plenty of clothes and I shouldn't be worried about a cardigan, but it was imprinted in my mind. And it worried me and I thought 'Gosh. Don't let it possess you. Please don't get obsessed over a cardigan'. I even asked, not Anna, I can't remember her name, the young lady at reception at the drop-in, because she lives down my road and I said 'Was the cardigan handed in?' and she said that if it was, it would be in the cupboard. But I didn't even leave it there I don't think. It was a total obsession. It worries me. It really does worry me.

I went to the hospital this morning to see the doctor and I saw Fran there. That's another client who goes to the drop-in. She was getting out of a cab. She was going to the day centre and she puts her arms round me and she said "Oh you" and I said "You are coming to Crumbs tomorrow?" We've got a group at Crumbs[12]. It's called 'Friends'. It did disband, but we're going to start it again and we'll go down tomorrow morning and have coffee and I said to Fran "You promise to come won't you" and she said "I will". And she's very low at the moment. She's very depressed. She's more than depressed really and she's got a lot of problems that's built up, that's caused it, you know, and I can totally …. my heart goes out for her really. I know her problems and my heart really does go out to her. To her as a person. She's a

---

[12] The drop-in centre Anne attends.

lovely person. It's nice to sit there and talk to about half a dozen ladies that have got my problems. We can relate to each other, you know. It's nice to be able to relate to somebody. They've all got problems and we all sit there and talk and we go out on day outings and things like that, you know. It's nice to be able to come in and somebody to say 'how are you today? Are you up or are you down?' *(laughs)*.

When I'm high I feel as if I could conquer the world. Then all of a sudden you've gone down and you're down in the hole again and you can't climb out of it. And you cry and you cry. But most of the time you cry alone. I think though, that the mental health services in general are very good. I think they do a marvellous job. I couldn't fault them, with what resources they've got. I mean, down here they're excellent, compared to London where I was. London hospitals have just gone down and down.

Amanda

Amanda was a thoughtful, quietly spoken and articulate young woman. She agreed to be interviewed in order to help and educate others about mental health difficulties. She lives with her partner in a house that they are in the process of renovating.

When I have been well I've found books a good resource in understanding others. Some books with long chapters are really difficult to read. But I found, you know, short stories or paragraphs easy to concentrate on. They can be quite inspiring, especially when you feel that you're not going to get better. I can feel like that quite often. That's why I wanted to talk to you really, to tell people that there is hope out there and that it is possible to move on.

I was admitted into a young person's psychiatric unit when I was fourteen but I'd say the problems started a year or two before that. I was an inpatient for a long time but I came out when I was about sixteen and I've managed to stay out. You know, sometimes hospital is the right place for you but sometimes it can be the wrong place. For recovery. I have had a few trips to A&E though.

I'm twenty-three now. In the psychiatric unit they said I had school phobia and anorexia. I didn't eat. I didn't drink water. I sometimes wonder whether it was anorexia.

In my mind, I just wanted to die. I wasn't allowed to kill myself so I would just not eat or drink.

The bad feelings started when I was about nine. There was a certain member of family who'd done things to me. And that gave me a bad feeling but it didn't start with the eating then. It didn't start with the eating until I was about thirteen. But it was when I was nine that something had happened and then, you know, at intervals between nine and thirteen, other things happened. A different variety. And then … *(pauses)* I think as my body started developing, I didn't like it anymore and I just stopped eating. I didn't want to be at home. So I stopped eating. Social workers got involved and psychiatrists and everything, but they didn't realise what was happening because I hadn't told anyone.

When I was going to school, I was passing out because I wasn't eating. The social workers came round to check out my home. Sometimes I think to myself, 'well they didn't do a very good job did they?' Which sounds awful because the social worker was lovely. My mum's also had a lot of problems, which contributed to things that I feel they could have spotted. Also when I was in the unit I never wanted to go home. They told me if I gained weight they'd let me home. Of course I wanted to lose even more, so I didn't have to go.

I was treated in the old, traditional ways; bed rest, no TV, no radio. The nurses were nice but that was depending on what I ate and whether I'd gained weight. If I'd lost weight then they weren't that nice. I'd have to lie down flat for half an hour after food. I was in an observation room where they used to watch me constantly through the window. But I didn't care. What did I think about? I thought about how life was ...(*pauses*) not nice. I felt I was being punished and so it just pushed me further into myself. If I ever wanted to hurt myself - if I ever mentioned it - it was straight away everything got taken off me. All my perks you know, my picture frames, pictures and books. So .... I think I learnt just to go into myself and not really say anything. I wasn't allowed to the toilet on my own, they would follow me. I understand they were doing it to keep me alive. I understand that. But I was just a mess.

I had psychiatrists. Every three months they'd change around. So they'd just get to know you and then they'd go. Or you'd just get to feel comfortable with them and then they're gone. Some of the other people in there I got to know eventually. Some really special friends. I don't really keep in contact with them today because I feel ...(*pauses*) maybe they want to, I don't know, get on with their lives or something. But to me, I did make special friends inside, who I could talk to and things.

When I was sixteen I became an outpatient. With regular appointments with a psychiatrist. I'd been in hospital for two years and it wasn't easy. As I started to develop, if men showed me attention, I reacted badly. It was then I'd mentioned to the psychiatrist that something someone was doing reminded me of stuff I didn't like from before.

I didn't really realise what it was all about until, until he said, "well, that's actually not right". Then things were just blown totally out of my control. The psychiatrist had told me that I'd be in full control, you know, of what happened next. But he immediately brought my parents in for a meeting and told them and then involved Social Services. I mean I know he was obliged, but there was very little talk to me and a lot of action going on. I went even more into myself. I felt so ashamed. Really ashamed. I couldn't look my parents in the eye. I didn't know what they were thinking of me, whether they thought I was lying, whether they thought I was bad and things. I'd never wanted them to know because they'd think I was so bad. And now they knew just like that.

They were shocked and surprised. They supported me as they thought best to, but I wouldn't say it always worked. About two weeks later I saw a birthday card written out on the bench top and it was to him. And I don't know, it just felt (long pause) …It caused a lot of ruptures in the family. They were told by the psychiatrist to treat me completely normally. The same as my two other sisters. I think in his eyes, it was to prevent me developing any problems but it really didn't work. It really compounded everything. I was just... *(pauses)*, I was just crying inside. A lot of the things I had to learn to deal with on my own, which my parents then saw as a threat, I think.

Like when I sleep at night, I have to have my door a finger width apart. I had to have my window open so I could escape if I needed to. I had a TV and mirror in my room and I had to cover them up. Completely cover them with paper because... not because of messages or anything, but because I felt he could watch me. He used to watch me a lot before and I felt he was looking at me through the TV and through the mirror. And the wardrobe. I used to have to pile loads of books in front of the wardrobe so it was difficult to open and close. He used to keep bad things in the wardrobe. I just used to be scared all the time. I knew that anyone in the family could just walk in the house at any time, because Mum and Dad still had contact with, you know, the family. Not with him though, apart from the birthday card. I did stuff to try and control things, control my fear. I couldn't have a shower with the mirror there, so I had to put a towel over the mirror. It felt as if he was still there looking at me through the mirrors when I took a shower.

All of these things I couldn't really tell anyone about. Eventually though I was referred to see an Occupational Therapist who I developed quite a good relationship with. She was really good and she was the only one who stopped and listened to me. I could tell her things like if I wanted to cut myself and she listened and didn't tell me off. Didn't alert everyone. I could tell her about wanting to die inside and she would listen and try to understand.

We also dealt with the effects of speaking up. The reactions of my family. How I was being treated at home. How Mum was becoming unwell so Dad's...all Dad's attention was going to Mum. To the point of, at one time, he asked me to move out because every time Mum saw me she couldn't bear it. It was really hard for my Mum because she's a twin, an identical twin. She'd always been really close to her twin and it was her twin's son who'd done those things. So it caused a separation there and a big family rift. It made her quite ill and at the time she blamed me. I was told that I'd torn the family apart, that I should have just kept quiet. Things like, 'Why don't you just move on? Leave it behind.' Every time I showed my feelings ... every time I tried to show emotion or feeling all I got back was frustration and anger.

I had a very close friendship with a male at this time. His family took me on board. They were lovely. They didn't tell me off for any of my behaviour and they listened. I used to go over very upset and sometimes I'd talk to my friend's mum and tell her things that had happened and then she'd tell me if it wasn't my fault. Inside I still thought it was.

I used to stay over there quite a bit. I had a bag of my stuff I used to keep there. I used to have to share a room with my friend. I didn't have a bedroom to myself or anything. Sometimes I'd go home and top up my bag and things. 'Cos I still officially lived at home... *(pauses)*, I used to feel very homesick a lot. Not for the home that was there but wanting to be part of a family with my mum and dad (*long pause*)...

I ended up getting into university with the help of my OT[13]. I don't remember much about being there when I look back. I know I focused on my work. I was really focused because that's all I could do. Everything was happening around me with my friends going out clubbing and drinking. It was all happening at Uni. And I was there, but not there. I was alongside it. It was good to be alongside it, better than being at home or living out of a bag. I still had a few eating problems there. I had support from a Special Needs Advisor in the department. I'd always put off going for help or

---

[13] Occupational Therapist.

support because of the way I'd been treated in the past. When I went eventually, they were very, very helpful.

I suffered, and still do, from very bad sleep. I find it very difficult due to my past. I feel like it's safer to sleep during the day. I can sleep during the day, which kind of knocks me around a bit. When everything goes quiet, I don't feel safe, I need noise. I can't sleep when it's all quiet. I don't know why.

I finished university somehow. I sat all my exams on my own, in a room, with extra time because I'm on medication as well, which affects concentration. I did all this, but every day I didn't want to live. I only did it because I was having to function. I was like a robot. On the outside I was functioning and Doctors would often say to me "well you must be okay because you're functioning". But on the inside I was dead. You feel like you're not functioning. Doctors and people, they're not always aware of that. They don't understand how you can function on the outside and not function on the inside. Each time, the better I got, they withdrew any help, rather than continuing to support me. They must have had their reasons I suppose.

I've found that you've really got to seek help and ask for it. Ask for it and also take it. A lot of the things I'm learning and dealing with are about accepting help. Although it's really hard to like accept things like a cuddle. You don't want to and you really push people away but it's the thing you're most longing for. You want people to hold you and tell you it's okay. For some reason you push people away but sometimes you've really got to just shut your eyes and allow that hug. Sometimes a hug can do wonder,s can work wonders.

I used to feel before that I shouldn't ask for help because of what would people think – I didn't dare - but then I felt I couldn't stand it anymore. Who cares what people think. I just need to feel better. In learning to ask for help I was able to stop with my anorexia. I managed to recover from that in about the last year of university. I knew I needed food. So three times a day I would eat. Even if I didn't want to. I just used to put it in my mouth and think well I must need it. I think I started to realise the effects it had on my body. I became aware of things, that I'd feel slightly better when I'd eaten. I'd got more energy to face things. I don't know exactly how I induced that. I wish I did because I would tell everyone. I think it comes with time. And with learning to ask for help.

After university I didn't want to go home. My friend, whose family had taken me on, had got a job down South and so I brought a bag down and stayed on his floor. I've been here ever since. I got a job as a bar person and I got registered with doctors here. And a psychiatrist. It didn't last long, me working. I just got ill. Worse and worse. I really deteriorated.

In my head, I never saw me completing a degree. So when I enrolled on the course, I didn't look ahead. I couldn't look beyond it, because there wasn't anything. I didn't think I'd still be here. And so when I finished I was lost. I really deteriorated ... I couldn't move out of bed. I was just waking up, soaking wet all the time, because of the sweat. I was tense all the time. Panicky. Shaky. Feeling suicidal all the time. You just don't want to live. People say 'but you're doing this and you've done that'. 'But I still want to die,' I'd think, 'I still don't want to be here'. That was such a strong feeling. I started drinking bottles of rum or something like that, with tablets. Then I met another friend who is my partner now. He used to sit with me sometimes. He never took me to the hospital because I used to beg him not to. I didn't want to go. An overdose? Yeah, several times. I used to be sick sometimes but he just used to sit and keep an eye on me. I asked him about it recently, I said, "How did you know that I'd be alright?". He said that he hadn't known.

The majority of my support and development came from my friends. And encouragement. You feel guilty at first, depending on them. Sometimes you need to depend on someone. You know, if things are so bad, you need to. I suppose in a way I did depend on my friends, but it wasn't in a negative way. It was in a way where I could depend on them and reach out when I needed them. And when I didn't, it didn't matter. Does that make sense? People say dependency is a bad thing but I feel that sometimes you need to depend on someone or something. There's a healthy dependency and that goes unrecognised. Unrecognised by mental health services as well.

I've found in my recovery I'm very much a person of three steps forward, two steps back, three steps forward, two steps back. I'm very much like that. I can really stride forward and feel really good. You can brush your teeth one day and it's easy. It sounds silly …but it doesn't take ages to get dressed. You can walk outside. Sometimes I'll breath in and hold my head high. I can feel really, really good. Then I'll come crashing down and I'll be back to - or at least I'll feel at that time - like I'm back to the beginning. I can't be though because now, although I still want to take the overdoses at points, I don't. You feel like you're back at the beginning; stage one, and that things will never get better again. Then you'll jump further forward than you had before. It's hard to understand it.

Unfortunately at the moment, I'm going through a bad patch and it seems to have been two weeks so far. And so I'm thinking, you know, 'how long is this going to take?'. But I suppose at least in the back of my mind I know what's happening. It is a bad patch. Sometimes the worse the bad patch is, the further you jump forward in feeling good. Maybe not good but different. You feel different. Better. I don't know what feeling good feels like. Does that sound strange? I think because I've been ill since my teens, when a lot of people learn their own feelings and values, at that time, well, I was in hospital. I didn't know what 'normal' feelings were. Now I think I'm kind of finding out about it them.

I get exhausted. When I'm feeling good I want to hold onto it and I will really push myself to stay there. I exhaust myself. And when I get tired and exhausted, that's when it all comes crashing in. Also, the time of the year makes a difference. The end of January was his birthday so I'm wondering if that was the cause of this last bout. Special occasions, family occasions, like when family used to meet up, at Christmas time and Easter time. Summer holidays when we'd go away on holiday together. It's times like that when it comes through. Sometimes you don't notice it and then it starts eating you up inside. Until it just consumes you completely and you don't know what to do with yourself. Like the other night, I was just pacing the bedroom. I've got a rug in there which is rippled up and down. I found that just walking on the rug with my feet, starting from toes and going to heel, massaged my feet and it was the only calming thing I could find. My partner looked at me, like 'what you doing?'. I was just pacing this rug and I was aware it was calming but to anyone else, they must have thought 'she's lost it'. It was just to get some feeling in my feet. It was the only feeling I could get to calm me. Sometimes I rock myself to sleep to try and calm my body and my thoughts. It can also depend on what I read. Sometimes I read things that can be triggering. I got a book recently, on Post Traumatic Stress disorder (PTS) actually. I was reading about other people but I saw flashes of my own life. I couldn't help it. Anyway I don't suppose its night-time reading, but of course I read it before I went to bed, so that didn't help me sleep.

I'm in touch with my family more now. I hadn't been for a while. I'd finally come to a point of where I'd stood up to them and said, "look, this is me, I've been through this and it's had an effect on me". Like it or lump it, in a way. Especially to my mum, who depended a lot on me on making her feel better. So I said "that's enough. I can't make you feel better. I need to think about me". My mum blew up, but I stood my ground. Since then everything's been a lot better. They understand that I find it difficult to go back to my hometown and so they'll come down to see me. I have no contact with outer family. It's too difficult.

My partner? We've had really intense patches. Very intense. A lot of it through him not understanding what it's like. I used to talk to him sometimes and tell him and he used to listen, but he didn't really understand. We've had our difficulties obviously, with the private part of our relationship. We've had difficulties there. We still do … *(pauses)*. I suppose in a way he's half partner, half carer. It sounds horrible but it's true. He comes home every day from work and gets me up. He gets me up and makes sure I'm okay. I do everything I can and when I can I do it myself. He knows I will. I'll fight to do that myself. But he will do it for me when I'm not well. Physically lift me up and make sure I get in the shower. He's on standby, he has his mobile kept on at work in case I need him. He's really supportive. I know he really loves me and for some reason I love him too and I didn't know I'd ever be able to feel that…. *(pauses)* He's taught me how to do a lot of outdoor stuff and to allow myself pleasures like having my rabbits. He knows I get a lot of happiness out of them.

Some of my behaviour can come across as childish to people. I don't fully understand it myself, but he just lets me get on with it. He lets me be me. At the same time, when I'm well I can give a bit back to him and I think he appreciates that. Which I think keeps it going really. So I'm not just permanently taking. I like to give him a lot back. He understands I can only do that when I'm well. I think what

I've found is you don't just have treatment and magically get better. It's all about working with it and working around things to make you feel better. Does that make sense?

I had, say two years off after Uni. and spent most of it in bed not well. As my friendship with my partner developed into a relationship, he started encouraging me more. I decided it might be wise to do things and I got a job. I did voluntary work at first. I went to the local job centre and asked for advice there and they were really supportive. If you go down the right avenues you can get the support. Don't just keep trying to battle on by yourself. At first I went to the usual desk and I was getting nowhere. They couldn't make head or tail of me. Then I got in with a Special Needs Advisor at the job centre and she completely knew what I was going on about and suggested voluntary work. So she got me set up with some voluntary work at the local volunteer centre. To begin with I'd really stress about having one hour a week there. Really stress about it. Say I did it on a Monday, on the Wednesday before, I'd start thinking about it. Working myself up to it. Going there was so hard. Just for one hour a week. Then I don't know how it happened but I was going in three days a week. You know, three mornings or three afternoons. Sometimes I'd joke with Robert (my partner) and say 'remember how I found it so hard to do one hour a week?' I think you have to keep on looking. People say to look towards the future but I've found that looking towards the past and seeing, well, look where I am now compared to then, helps me a lot. It spurs me on a lot. I know when Robert encourages me, that really spurs me on. I suppose part of my personality is out to please people. Which is a good and a bad thing. When it's healthy, it's good.

So I was doing voluntary work and eventually I felt ready to go into paid work. I just walked into a chemist one day and asked about a job they had advertised in the window and they said okay. Of course, I don't sleep during the night, but I managed to turn up every morning. I did that for about four months. When I was strong and okay it was good, but when I started, if nightmares and things had affected me, you know, I'd have bad days and there was no support at work. They had no understanding. I started to really struggle with their attitude towards me. When I first went there, I just blurted out, "I've been off for the last two years because I haven't been very well, but I'm ready to get back into work now and focus on getting better." I just came out with it because I didn't know any other way round it. So they were fully aware of my problems. It's good that they'd taken me on and given me the chance. I think what happened in the end was they were too pushy. They didn't want any of my emotions or anything. They just wanted me to function and perform. Which usually I'm quite good at, but when your emotions get too much you just can't. I lasted it about four months and then I just deteriorated again. They weren't working with me. They were working more against me. If people work with you, you can do loads and achieve, but when they just work alongside or against you, you just get nowhere.

I went to the job centre and saw the Special Needs Advisor and told her about the situation I was in. I really was not well at the time. I told her some things that had been said to me and she told me about a programme where they can come in and assess the situation and try and help. She got in touch with the chemist, but they were having none of it. So I made a decision that I didn't want to work at a place if they weren't going to be open and you know, try and work with me.

Then it was back to voluntary work. I was quite down in the dumps. I applied for loads of jobs. Then I got set up with an agency where if you've been out of work for a while, they can help you get back in. They can help you with application forms and interviews and things. So I got a job coach and I did my application forms. Luckily they help identify what areas you needed help in. With me I can fill out forms but it's the emotions and the facing people I have difficulty with. The social side. I went to some interviews on my own and didn't get the jobs because they said I was too - you know, that my application form was good but I obviously couldn't handle the social part of the job. My job coach came along to an interview with me so she could examine where I was going wrong. That was with a mental health organisation working on a telephone support line. I got it! She didn't need to assess me after all.

Working there has opened my eyes a lot to what it's actually about. You don't get told what it's about. You don't realise that there are people out there who understand. There aren't people out there who can change your life with a magic wand or a miracle cure. But there are people out there. People who understand and listen. They don't see you as different, they understand you as a person, and will go alongside you, work with you. Somehow, I think that understanding and acknowledgment is quite a feel-good factor.

I've had loads of support since I started working and I'm working three days a week now, eight hour shifts. I've been doing that for five months. I had to come home once because I was really ill, mentally. They were fine with that. Other than that I've had one day off because I couldn't face it but that's all. Not bad going really. Just by people working with you and listening.

And through talking. Completely just coming out with it, saying it and being honest. So long as it's a receptive person who'll listen and try to help you. Sometimes if I ever want to hurt myself, if I can say it and tell someone and they listen and acknowledge it, the feeling goes and I don't need to do it. I can talk about things with my line managers. I feel I could say it to the people that I work with as well, but I don't want to at the moment. We're already in quite a pressured job. If I ever felt desperate, then they would be there, but I don't want to put that extra pressure on them. But they are aware. The people who I work with are aware about the way I am. They don't make anything of it, but they accept it. It's just me.

It helps me to understand things when I listen to callers. Listening to them helps put me in perspective. I'm really interested in other people and their perceptions and it's helped me to learn. Before I only had a view of my perception of the abuse. Working there you get the story of the mother, the father, the daughter. You get all of them ringing up and talking and so you get the different perspectives. Sometimes I think to myself, I've never thought of it in that way before. I never say that down the phone to them though. I treat each call for it's own sake. I listen and I never disclose personal things about myself. I know I could if I wanted to but I just feel personally, it's not somewhere I want to go. I'd rather be there for them, because in the past I have had people, you know, doctors tell me about their children and personal stuff. But I'd rather be there for that person who needs me. When you talk to someone who's really frantic and at the end of a call they're feeling really positive, you come off feeling really, really good. Sometimes I come off smiling. I do... I do have some problems there. Sometimes it can be a very similar situation to mine and it becomes a problem if it's too much. It's good for me to an extent, but sometimes if it's too... or perhaps, if I have a flashback and it triggers my own thoughts too much, it's a problem. I've learnt how to monitor myself better now and if I feel I'm not going to be okay, I just don't take that call. If I'm feeling strong, I'll take it.

Although I'm in a completely comfortable work place, I do struggle. You struggle with what people will think of you. They might all think positive and good things, but you still have doubt sometimes. I know that sounds strange. I just hope that I'll be able to develop more and become more confident. My aim is to be working full time and have a busy, active life. At the moment I stay in and I go to work and that's it. I've found though...I've found for me to be able to do things, I need to slow down and I've found that to cope with work, I needed to allow myself to slow down for a bit.

Now that I'm aware of everything that's available and that I'm more able to recognise the things that are helpful to me, I'm going to ask for some actual treatment for Post Traumatic Stress Disorder. I've read up and there are actually lots of treatments out there. I've never had any treatment for the main cause of things. With how to deal with my flashbacks and what to do when they happen and stuff. So I'm going to actually request someone. There are people out there who know about it and I want to work with someone who does.

I get a lot of pleasure out of greenery. Green trees. I also get a lot from my rabbits. They give me a lot of love. I get a lot out from sitting in the garden. I force myself to go for walks. I never want to go but then I go and I always feel better afterwards. Even if it's one foot in front of the other and that's all I can do, just plod, I feel better afterwards. Or being dumped in the shower. Sometimes that works. Or dumped in the bath. I suppose you wash things away a bit. I'm still on medication for depression, on quite high doses. Sometimes I wonder if it's actually depression I've got and I don't think it is. I think I'm experiencing an effect of my past, which is quite normal really. It's a normal reaction. But then to society my behaviour seems abnormal.

I do some creative things. When I'm feeling okay and can concentrate I like to do some crosswords and that takes me away from myself. I like to read too. I always set myself really little goals because if I think to myself I'll do this, this and this today, then I'll panic and I can't do any of it. So I say I'll just start doing this and see how far I can get.

Usually I end up finishing it. Eventually you'll start doing it and before you know you've done it. It's not so hard.

Eileen

Eileen has lived for most of her life in Zimbabwe but moved to England in February 2002. She was an incredibly positive, smartly dressed woman eager to talk to as many people as possible about mental illness and its effects. She works as a volunteer at a 'Save the Children' shop, where she says she enjoys meeting and engaging with people.

I am one of seven children. My mother had a child by her first marriage. My father had two surviving triplets and then my parents were married and they produced my twin and I. Beg your pardon, twin and *me*, and my sister, my younger sister and my brother Harry.

My twin and I were the only ones who inherited mental illness from my mother. She was psychotic, but in those days they didn't seem to know the conditions, so what she was precisely, I don't know. Which is why I'm here (in London) this week, to find out how one illness can develop into two differing illnesses.

She was either schizophrenic or manic-depressive. I'm schizophrenic and my twin is manic-depressive. We all came out of our childhood with considerable success, we were poor but we had a good schooling and I was head girl at school. I went on to do my University degree *(pauses)...* I think I must condense this a bit. It wasn't until I was 34 until after I married my first husband that I developed schizophrenia. It was triggered by our bankruptcy. That was a stress factor. It was also a greatly unhappy marriage. However, I'm very grateful that I didn't develop the illness in my teens because not only was I able to get a training but also I was able to develop a career before I became ill. I'm a French teacher and I did train to do Latin but it was dropped from the curriculum in Rhodesia. After my second marriage, I also taught in primary school for nine years.

I met my husband (my first one) when I had my first teaching post. I met him in Rhodesia. I was very naive and I was very quickly impregnated *(laughs)*. Instead of continuing with my teaching I followed him to Salisbury, which is a city in Rhodesia and he agreed to marry me. But there was no love on his part. Although our marriage lasted for thirteen years, it was not a happy marriage. In the course of things I had three children and then I happily got divorced *(laughs)*. Prior to my divorce, I with my schizophrenia, was able to go back to teaching despite being hospitalised for nearly a year.

I'm so grateful for the fact that there wasn't any ham-stringing legislation in Rhodesia that stopped you from being forcibly hospitalised and allowed you to be retained in hospital until you were better. Even then I was heavily sedated and my early teaching wasn't very distinguished.

Eventually I decided I would give up my medication and I stockpiled ten months supply of tablets, took them back to my psychiatrist and said to him, 'I don't need these, you can have them back again' and he took me by the hand and said 'well done. Some people don't need them.' But that didn't prove to be the case because about two years later, I became once again manic and hyperactive.

I've just had an interview this morning with Dr Kuzeli exploring the nature and origins of my illness. He concluded that although I had disorder of the thinking process/processes and various delusions, I didn't have any hallucinations, I didn't feel I was being governed by some external force, I didn't have any weird sensory perceptions and I didn't hear voices. 'Um ... *(pauses)* so he says I'm probably manic. However all my psychiatrists in Harare and in Salisbury agreed I was schizophrenic and I've certainly responded to the medication.

So in 1980, I was hospitalised again. At that time I had become involved with a group of Pentecostals. They had told me that my illness was due to demonic possession and that you're supposed to cast demons out. So once again I decided to give up the medication. In fact every time the doctor said that they were keeping the dose low so I could go back to work, I ended up giving up the medication and there were about three relapses in succession until they

143

finally kept me in hospital for a long time. Then they released me; very comatose and very fat, and I went to stay with my cousin who was a happy-clappy. By that time I finally realised that I had to take my medication. I managed to lose the weight by dieting and they put me on this wonderful drug called Orappimozide[14]. At the end of '82, I was pronounced by the medical board as fit for work again and that really was the beginning of my life. Not only was I able to function properly without any side-effects but I also began to perfect my career and I began to teach in earnest and with some success. And during that period - eight years - I remained on Orap and during that period I met my second husband and subsequently my lover when my husband died *(laughs)*.....But then in '92, I could no longer get Orap', it was not obtainable in Rhodesia anymore, so my Doctor put me back onto Largactil. I still worked, I still managed to teach but I lost all my vivacity, and creativity, and conversation, my conversational ability and became fat again. As Zimbabwe plunged into disaster, it became harder and harder for me to get out because the inflation was so great and my income wasn't meeting my needs. You couldn't get cars so I had no mode of travel. And my medication...Finally my landlord managed to get a supply of Orap for me and my son who had left Zimbabwe also sent me a supply from England and I managed also to import

---

[14] Hereon referred to as 'Orap'.

some. But of my income of $23000 a month, my medication was costing $20 000. So when my lover married somebody else who was also of my vintage *(laughs)*, I finally accepted my children's invitation to come to England. Since my first husband had been British, I had a British passport *(pauses)*…I'm now living in Weybridge because my two sons are there and it has been the happiest time of my life. I like to tell everybody that life begins at sixty *(laughs)*. I've joined a mental health centre in Weybridge because I wanted everybody else who suffers from mental illness to experience the same quality of life that I do.

Also something I vainly wish for, is that people with mental illness could be employed. I've applied for three jobs since I've been here. I'm a teacher and when I first arrived I applied for supply teaching but after observing the local schools, I decided that after spending five years in a college without discipline in Harare, I wouldn't repeat that experience in government schools. So I applied for a job in a fish and chip shop, a job in the bakery and in the Spar shop and I was accepted for none. So I said to the manager of Spar, I said 'Will you please tell me if my application is rejected, whether it's because of my age or my 'emit' status'. Do you know the word 'emit'? It means outsider, foreigner *(laughs)*. He said 'No, it's because you're overqualified.'

John Nash who features in '*A Beautiful Mind*' - I've read the book - is supposed to have gone off medication in his late seventies. I would like to know what his record is when he hits his deathbed. And if there's anybody else, who's been for a prolonged time, say more than two years off medication, I would like to speak to them and meet them.

The biggest disadvantages are the side-effects of these medications, of these new and old anti-psychotics. But as I say with Orap, I have not a single side-effect but I have with Largactil. I've never been in hospital in England. My last hospitalisation was in '82, in Harare, and I haven't needed to be hospitalised since. I've been stable for twenty years.

Initially when I became ill, my first husband was very dismissive of me. Although in the divorce I got custody, when I became ill again obviously he had to take the children. After coming out of hospital the second time, I went round to visit my children and he said: 'Have nothing to do with your mother. Can't you see she's mad?'
He has always anticipated that I would remain mad forever and is now quite surprised. He is also living near Weybridge and he has seen me recovered and I think he's beginning to alter his viewpoint. He's recently said to me as other people have said, both patients and outsiders; 'What are you involving yourself with mental health for, you're alright, why

bother about anybody else?' That's from patients and *(pauses)*... from the sane public. I do it because I know what it is like to be mentally ill. I know how horrible it is, and I don't want anybody else to go through that experience and stay ill, or to bear the side effects that they have to tolerate.

In Zimbabwe when I first became ill, the government continued to employ me. They knew of my mental illness yet they still employed me and when I became ill again they continued to pay my salary while I was hospitalised and while I was recuperating. Nevertheless I didn't divulge my illness to everybody. It was only a small circle of intimate friends who knew, just to be on the safe side. I had to work, not teaching the pupils but also meeting the parent body, so in fact I did like to keep it under wraps. But fellow sufferers who were my friends, all managed to get employment, so there was far less discrimination against mental illness in Zimbabwe, than there is here in England. Since I've been in England I've made it my policy to be quite open about my illness. My younger brother says to me, 'You shouldn't do that, you should wait until you've known your friends for about twenty years and then they can see that you're OK!' But I haven't got twenty years! *(laughs)* I said, 'It's alright, you don't have to worry, I don't divulge it until it becomes a natural conversational point.' Mostly I've had a good reception of this disclosure but 'er *(pauses)*...there have been some notable exceptions to that.

My son-in-law took me up to Bude to visit his mother's cousin, to some sort of party. I chatted for quite some time quite flirtatiously with one man there and I said, 'Incidentally you know, I'm a schizophrenic' and then he clammed up. Clammed up. Stood up and went over to the other side of the room, sat down and refused to speak to me again.

When I'm in my son's shop he says, 'You mustn't tell people you're schizophrenic because you'll antagonise customers'. He's got a cyber café. But it's amazing when you disclose this fact to find how many people either directly or indirectly know of mentally ill people. Lots of people have got a friend or relative or something with it.

One person of note, whom I thought had an understanding as she was well-educated - is well-educated - and she was married to a pharmacologist, said to me one day, 'Oh you must stop talking about mental illness. It should be swept under the carpet' she said. So I ceased to frequent the shop where she works and found other people I can talk to. I've just become secretary of the Osteoporosis Society of Cornwall; I've told the chairman and his wife all about my schizophrenia, and the other people there, and it seems that generally the more intelligent the person, the more open-minded they are. The more educated, the more enquiring. The music appreciation group, I've told them and they don't bat an eyelid.

I'm telling people - I'm doing it - I'm telling people because I want to educate the public and the policy of simply handing out leaflets once a year will give the public no instruction whatsoever. They need to see the patient in a recovered state, functioning normally for them to overcome this attitude or prejudice that they have. The popular idea that schizophrenics are all violent and nasty, well that's certainly not true (long pause)...

My brother, my twin, did in fact get ill three years before me. He was in the RAF when he got ill and they boarded him. He was having such a hard time that he went back to Zimbabwe and he's worked since he's been back. He's always had jobs, he worked as a taxi driver in London for a while. On certain occasions over the years, he's had the whim to give up his lithium. With dire consequences. Mad as a hatter again. For now he takes it. I did wonder about my daughter for a while but I think she's alright. I think my sons have also passed the deadline because I was thirty-four when I became ill, and they are thirty-six and thirty-eight, so I think they've gone past the danger mark. But who knows whether my grandchildren are susceptible to it? My daughter's got twin daughters.

I don't miss Zimbabwe, not one jot. The only thing I regret is that my friends and relatives were left behind in that shambles. I don't miss the climate, the English climate doesn't bother me in the least. I've got this sort of inner contentment now and it's so wonderful to live in a civilised country. One thing I really value is the library network. Also in Zimbabwe I could never ever have afforded a computer or had access to one. Now with my son's help I've become or rather I am, in the process of becoming computer literate. And with the internet of course, I've maintained contact and expanded my contacts. And revived old friendships.

I get Income Support and I don't take it for granted. I don't wish to bleed the state. Just this last week I volunteered to go and work in one of the charity shops. And I budget very carefully. I record everything. Everything. My greatest area of expenditure is the telephone *(laughs)*. Also because there's this fantastic availability of charity shops, I've been able to kit myself out for next to nothing. This skirt is a charity shop acquisition – a couple of pounds. Shoes, one pound.

I've never heard voices. Never heard them. One thing that did happen to me; when I became born again, manically born again was that I received the gift of talking in tongue. Now that I can look at it objectively, I can see that it is no more that gobbledy-gook. But that stuck with me for quite a while after I'd recovered. Especially if I was undergoing any form of mild stress or agitation, I would just lapse into this tongue. It must have been pure habit because it's completely gone now.

The advice I would give to fellow sufferers is that when you're hospitalised and you're advised not to give up your medication, don't. You may feel horrible, you may feel dreadful but bear with it. On the coach coming to London, I wrote a poem in which I said, 'Bite down hard on the bullet', meaning be patient, and ride the bad side effects. Let your psychiatrists alter your dosage until you're well. Don't on any account give up the medication. If necessary ask your doctor to experiment with other medications until you can find the optimum one. If you're on the right drug, as I was when I was put on Orap', you will be able to lose weight and you will be able to concentrate again. I mean even when I was on Largactil, I still managed to teach. I wasn't inspired, I wasn't lively but I still managed to earn a living. I wasn't even really that tired, except when I first came out of hospital, when I was discharged for the very first time. In that state I couldn't even cross the road. Couldn't negotiate my way around a supermarket but eventually my sense of self came back because the dose was diminished.

I've only been married whilst ill once, the first time . After which I was very happily divorced! With my second marriage, I was only married from February to June in '87 because my husband had a heart attack. He didn't believe I was schizophrenic because I was so normal, so creative. Since then I've had relationships but I've never remarried.

I never go through bad days. I try to say to people I meet who are going through a bad patch, 'I don't have bad days'. If I have a little minor setback of circumstances and I get a bit down, it's not really depression, it's just a knock - it won't last for more than half a day, or even a couple of hours. Then I'll spring back to normal.

Everyday I get out of bed with a feeling of anticipation and joy. I said to the pharmacist, the one who sent me some Orap' from England, I said 'If I die at least I've had a good spell of living'. You see since I've been here, I've been told that one of the possible side effects of Orap' is Cardiac Erythema. I hadn't known about that but I'm afraid I'm going to gamble with it, because I'm on such a low dosage, I only take 1mg, twice a day and the quality of life I enjoy on it makes it a worthwhile gamble.

My doctor in Harare said to me, 'To what do you attribute your recovery?, Your stabilization?' I said, 'Because I've never had it easy'. I've had a hard life and it's made me resilient. I also think that my training as a teacher has made me very resilient and organised. I take my medication methodically, and if I've offered advice to people, well, it's been that they should examine themselves; note down these side effects and difficulties. Try to be of sterner stuff. Not to feel sorry for themselves. There are far worse physiological conditions and mental illness is just a physiological condition, it's an imbalance in the brain...I would hate to have arthritis or...MS...or...or...at least mental illness can be controlled.

Experiences which people want to see as a cause are merely triggers. Triggers. I don't know about depression. I was trying to discuss depression with the doctor this morning, because I know someone who is depressed. I said, 'Is it a chemical thing, the origin of depression?' I know very little about depression. Certainly with manic depression and schizophrenia, it's a chemical imbalance. Of course the triggers can vary immensely. As can the personality of the individual sufferers and the fact that you can get gentle, loving schizophrenics and violent, nasty ones is just a manifestation of these personalities.

The thing I find frustrating is that patients here won't talk although I'm getting used to that now. I'm used to talking to fellow patients in Zimbabwe but there's... *(pause)* there's this great cloud of confidentiality here that shrouds everything. I met a man whose wife is mad in Weybridge, she's either schizophrenic or manic depressive but they won't tell him, her husband, what condition she has. Which to me is totally stupid. I find it frustrating and some of the patients either don't know what they're suffering from or refuse to discuss it and talk instead about labels. Well to me, every physiological condition has to have a label, in order for it to be treated. In a mental health magazine I read recently it said, 'Schizophrenia is an ugly label'. But the label is merely a name. The ugliness doesn't come from the name, the ugliness comes from not only those who condemn it, like the public, but also from psychiatrists, who encourage this idea of caginess. We mustn't, mustn't give it a name. There should be more frank openness about it and I find it much less like this in Zimbabwe. It's something I'm still trying to figure out, what has happened in England? To me, the thing that seems to be the factor is the excessive preoccupation with human rights. The fact is that the rights of a child has ruined the education system, has arrogated the child, over his parents and teachers. The fact that patients have the right to discharge themselves from hospital 'um – I've lost the thread – yes, these rights, well it hasn't penetrated the mental health legislation in Zimbabwe. Nobody says the patient has the right to determine their own treatment. They leave that to the discretion of the psychiatrists.

Also, there's less care and protection of the mentally ill in Zimbabwe. They have to fight to survive and I think that's a very good thing. It toughens them up, develops their skills, gives them a greater sense of meaning and direction. There was one particular young man who was in hospital when I was first ill, he was a flutist, he had his flute in hospital and he also was an actor and a poet. When he left hospital he went into the media and now does a lot of media work and advertising. Another girl I was with, she was also a manic-depressive, she was a teacher and she went on to be head in a couple of schools of the infant department. Denise, a religious one was extremely creative and artistic. She didn't need to work because her husband was well-to-do.

England is fantastic in its' provision. Especially for those, who perhaps are so severely ill that they never overcome their symptoms. I mean I will never be able to repay what they've done for me and with my medication. Also the social security is fantastic. It's just these two facts really, especially that they won't employ the mentally ill. The other one is the refusal of patients to take medication. The fact that they are being aided and abetted in that decision. In Rhodesia, in Zimbabwe, *we* called sectioning, committal. I was committed both in my first illness and in my second bout of illnesses. Nobody told me that I should question I and I didn't. Have I got my point across?

I recently read the work of a psychiatrist called Roy Porter. I enjoyed that very much. Not only the historical aspect but his attitude to mental illness. He didn't go in for all sorts of euphemisms. It's as if people shouldn't use the word mad nowadays. He said they even use the phrase 'mad with love' *(laughs)*. When you are mad there's no other description for it, you're totally mad, insane *(laughs)*. Amongst the other euphemisms is service-user. You can't use the word patient and yet 'patient' only means that you're suffering.

Patients must take their medication, not only for their own sake but also because when you develop a mental illness for which you don't ask, there is no fault or shame. Many patients seem to be ashamed of it. You've done nothing wrong, unlike the obese who overeat, they (the ill patients) must do it for the sake of the whole body of sufferers worldwide. To promote a positive image. You must realise that you've got to do your utmost to get better.

But I can see that if there is no prospect of a job, where's your motivation? Where's your direction? And I haven't found many - except for this one depressed man, whom I've befriended - who have an enquiring mind. This is just locally of course. There's no spirit of enquiry. The daycentre isn't stocked with reference material, I haven't seen any mental health magazines there. There should be loads of information available to the patient. I've got all the books I've read from the library. There's so many opportunities, even supposing you can't get a job, you can still extend yourself, make life interesting.

Sometimes it's difficult. I recently joined a creative writing class. It was a part of U3A, which stands for university of the third age, for retired people. There's one particular man who disapproved of me, he took an instant dislike to me. At one meeting, when I eventually got it out of him, he said, that in the first place, I was too highly educated for the group. In the second my accent was too thick, so he couldn't understand me. In the third place he said I kept talking about schizophrenia and mental illness. Fourthly, he thought that because I am so curious about everything, that that was a sign of my metal illness. I'm still going to it but I have to give it up anyway because it clashes with my new commitment to the charity shop. But it's alright, I can write by myself, I don't need a group to do my writing.

I love music. Good music. Not popular music. In fact it's why joined the music appreciation group. Although I've never received any instruction in classical music, it's like a physical experience to listen to good music. It penetrates you. Woos you. It's far more calmative than doing a series of exercises or meditations.

I haven't seen that many films – I think I've seen two films since I've been here. In England. I didn't see many films in Harare either because I had transport difficulties. Although I have seen films on television. I haven't got a television now and I read a lot. I've always tended to read non-fiction rather than fiction but I'm now able to catch up on some novels, historical novels that I had missed. I'm presently reading Gulliver's Travels which I never, ever got round to reading.

Everyday my first base is my son's cyber cafe, where I download my e-mail. I make it my business to help my sons as much as I can, so I help my son around the shop with the menial tasks. I don't know much about the stock *(laughs)* but I help make sure his shop is clean and organised. I make a daily visit to the charity shops, though I'll have to call a halt to that soon because I'm becoming over-equipped! Then there's usually something on, like one of my activities, the creative writing or music appreciation and I've also been to a couple of computer classes. I go to the library sometimes to receive instruction and I've become more acquainted with my laptop. I'm also working on my book, it's about my life, with a view to encouraging other mental patients.

My most lonely times are in the evenings and weekends because my sons are involved with their own lives. On Orap, I'm so gregarious and garrulous that I do like to converse with people. I enjoy talking to people. Of all the people with whom I'm friendly with on a conversational basis, very few have responded to my invitation to visit. I said, in one circular letter that I sent; that I had learned long ago that the English were very reticent about hospitality unlike the Rhodesians who entertain with camaraderie. I said, 'If an Englishman's home is his castle, then why pray, do some raise the drawbridge and clang shut the fort gate?'

My relationship with my sons is good. My youngest son says I mustn't correct people's grammar. Once I spoke to a schoolboy near the supermarket, a big fat boy, whose shirt was hanging out, as they all are *(laughs)*, I said on impulse, 'Tuck your shirt in. It's very untidy.' So Richard said to me 'If you do that mother you're going to get mugged one of these days.' Andrew says I mustn't talk to his clients because I intimidate them with my vocabulary. I still do, of course. But I do get on with my sons. It's my daughter whom, who's become a bit estranged from me. I think she's still got the negative image of me when I was on Largactil *(pauses)*...

On the one hand she I am so vain, then the other she's got a very poor image of me *(pauses)*... When I first arrived at Gatwick, they met me at the airport and they put me up for a week. One of the first things she said to me was 'Mother, if you don't do something about your teeth, you'll never get a job because it will jeopardise your interview.' Then she says to me, 'You're so self absorbed'. Well I think to some degree everybody is self-absorbed, and I'm not selfish. I'm involved with lots of people and lots of things. At one stage when I phoned her, she would be very curt and abrupt...(*long pause*) 'Um but then I have, all sorts of...well, I have re-established with so many people who give me positive feedback. I'm hoping that she's just going through a difficult time, with young children. She lacks for nothing material so I don't know why she should be so discontent...(*pauses*).

At weekends if my sons are free we might go out somewhere. I've been to two beaches since I've come here. I rely upon my sons to take me places though. I could catch the bus and travel where I please but I don't want to go to places by myself. In my opinion it's not where you go, it's whom you go with *(laughs)*. I'm such a curious person, I like to make observations about things and I like to share them with people.

Craig

I met Craig at a drop-in centre he sometimes attends. Then, and subsequently he was dressed in army camouflages. If he was trying to blend into the background he failed because his friendly and engaging manner made him stand out. Craig writes poetry and studies philosophy in his spare time. He lives with his mum in Bristol.

I think I've always been ill. The voices go back almost as far as I do. They were there when I was little. I was ill then. I've heard them for as long as I can remember. I've always had really vivid dreams and nightmares and stuff too. Let me tell you about the nightmares I had when I was younger. One nightmare was like, well, there was a labyrinth, it was pitch black in this labyrinth, you couldn't see anything. There was this thing chasing me through this labyrinth. Coming up behind me you know. Getting louder and louder and I was running as fast as I could but I was running into a dead end. So I turned and ran in the other direction and this kept going on and on and on. Me running and it right behind me. I used to have that one quite a lot.

Another one I had a lot was to do with those spinning toys that you used to get. The ones where you'd plunge the handle down and it would spin round and round really fast. I used to dream about me making it go faster and faster and faster until it went so fast it exploded and all the colours from this spinning top went right across my field of vision. That one used to wake me up. I used to wake up crying to that. I think maybe it was to do with limitations. I always wanted to *be* the spinning top going faster.

I suppose at some point I must have realized that I couldn't get strong enough or go fast enough and that there were limitations to me. I think that's where the dreams came into it. I think both of those dreams had something to do with that.

I used to have imaginary friends when I was little. Well actually they were imaginary enemies. They used to curse me all the time. Cuss is a better word perhaps. But they used to swear at me and call me derogative names and all of that. In them days I used to ignore them and they sort of like faded away over the years but then I started doing drugs and they came back again. But when they came back it was a more spiritual experience. I was more able to comprehend them.

Anyway when I was older people started noticing that I was becoming ill. They couldn't not do really. I started painting strange symbols on my bedroom walls and smashing mirrors and setting fire to bins because I thought they were full of magical spells. Yeah, I went a bit weird. That's not the half of it though, you know. I went a bit weirder than that. I used to walk around the countryside, like in Autumn. All I had on was a string jumper and a pair of trousers and that was about it. Barefoot and everything. That was completely barmy. I used to walk down the middle of the road, rather than on a pavement because roads were like scars on the skin of the earth. And if you'd walk down the middle of them, it wouldn't make them worse. It was a bit weird that was. That didn't last very long. I had to stop, people were like taking too much notice of me. I was getting horns beeped at me and stuff. I was walking around barefoot out of respect for the earth. You couldn't wear shoes. It's a bit weird, all potty stuff, I've put it all to one side. It's all madness now. I was 23 then.

I was, I was…there was a time I was trying to speak like…oh it was weird. I read down the alphabet and I was rolling the letters over my tongue, like 'Aahh', 'Ber', 'Cuh' and I tried making a language out of the sounds, trying to put a meaning to each sound. Basic ape man type of thing. That's to give you an example of how mad I was because I thought it could be a universal language that hadn't been discovered yet.

I've always had this illness but not always in the same context. Like I said when I was a kid it was mainly abusive words. And I can remember a voice in my head saying, 'Do you remember what you've gotta do for us?'. Of course I didn't, you know. I hadn't got a clue.

The good thing about my schizophrenia is that I've been able to get benefits from it you know. Although it's very, very abusive and horrible and all that, I've managed to salvage my religion out of it. I've managed to get that out of my madness. So for me it's worth it, to have gone through it. There are benefits. Needless to say I'm not a Christian. I did go to a Vicar once though. What did he tell me? I think he just said 'Go away'. 'Cos I was going on about snakes and stuff. It's like heresy isn't it really? Perhaps if I was a good Christian then he would have listened to me but I was some - what do they call them - atheist is it? And I was mad to boot.

My religion is difficult to describe. I've written it all down. I've written poems about it. All my poems are from my serious side, my religion and all that. If you look through them, you'll probably be able to make some sense of what I'm saying. To me everything is magic; you know the sun, the planet, the leaves. I'm not saying it's a lie, I'm just saying it's magic. I mean scientists they try to explain things scientifically and religious people, they try to explain everything supernaturally. To me they're all part of the same thing, magic.

I wasn't happy at school. I was really good and I was really clever but I remember the very first time I went to infant school my mum had to carry me because I wouldn't go. I was like that for a few weeks. I was kicking and screaming and punching at her while she carried me to school. Eventually that stopped but it sums up my general feeling of school really. I just didn't like it.

We did our 11 plus at junior school and then we went to the comprehensive. I did really well and was in the highest class. Nobody from my junior school was in that school and I got really disillusioned and started doing things wrong on purpose and all that sort of stuff so they sent me down a class because I was disruptive *(laughs)*.

I started mixing with more disruptive people and this one guy said to me, 'Well if you don't like sports, why don't you just skive off.' So I did and I enjoyed it. And then I thought, 'well hang on, I don't like chemistry either', so I skived off that. Then it was religious education. Eventually I ended up missing the entire last year of school. I didn't even go in one day.

Then it moved on into work. I got this little motorbike and all I wanted to do was just ride around on it. So I didn't get a job for ages. The only reason I got a job was because they threatened me, they said 'If you don't get a job we're stopping your dole money'. So I got a job for about 9 months. I was working in a chrome-plating factory. I got a new motorbike, a 250cc thing when they were legal for 17 year olds or whatever it was. You could ride it on L-plates. I rode it to work and there was this guy there and he had exactly the same type of bike. He said, 'I'll give you a race home'. So I said 'OK' and I had an accident. The very first day I got it. It was quite a close call. I was very lucky. When I was in there (the hospital) first of all, they said 'Look, it's 50/50 chance of survival'. They said that to me mam, you know, and she obviously got really freaked out by that. She doesn't like me having motorbikes *(laughs)*. No mother likes them do they? But then about three days later they threw me out. Said there was nothing wrong with me.

Anyway my motor biking, well, I never had the money to put the thing right, so I started stealing motorbikes. That didn't help. Fortunately, I've got over all this you know, I don't do it anymore. I'm a dedicated pedestrian now. It's better really, you know, for the health thing and also you don't get caught in traffic jams. You don't let loads of carbon monoxide into the atmosphere. It's pretty good really. There's nothing wrong with it. I reckon the population of England ought to be given a pushbike.

Eventually I started nicking with these people that smoked cannabis and all that. And this guy, I was friendly

166

with, a mate, said he needed money to get loads of hash and LSD and stuff. He didn't have any way of getting the money, so he said 'Look, you flog your motorbike and I can guarantee you'll get twice as much money back in a matter of weeks and you can go and get another one. So we did and basically we blew the drugs in about 5 hours. It was like non-stop getting high...(*pauses*)

I spent the next 5 years getting stoned. And then I spent the next twenty years mentally ill. Well, like diagnosed mentally ill, you know. I weren't just getting stoned then, I was getting paid for being disabled and getting stoned. Then, about 5 years ago I gave up drinking and smoking and all sorts. I started to get these pains in my chest a lot. So that's why I stopped really. I don't get them anymore. And I never really liked drink anyway. Didn't like the taste of it or nothing. I sort of like, just woke up to it as well. The thing is, it depends on the people you mix with as well. Since I've been diagnosed as being mentally ill like, since I've heard all these voices and since I've actually spoken about them - when I was a kid, I didn't used to talk about them, you know - but since you know I've been an adult they've become very spiritual to me. And I do talk about them because I think it's something that should be shared with people. All my friends though, they disappeared, one after the other, right. It was like my spiritual experience was their pain in the backside. They didn't want to know. They all disappeared. I know it's very cynical, but I don't believe in friends anymore. I just don't think there are any. I know it sounds really cynical but that's how I see it really. I don't mind really. I think I'm a bit more sure of myself now, of where I'm going and that. I'm a bit more clear in my mind, less confused by all these other people.

The thing is though, like, I attend different groups and centres and all that. And like I say I don't believe in friends and I don't really want 'em, but the reason I go to these groups is because if I didn't mix with people, then I'd go totally barmy. But I haven't got any friends so I've *got* to go to these groups and mix with people. It's very important. It's very important to, 'cos if you're mad, you've got to be able to see what's not so mad around you, you know. It's like you don't walk into walls because you can see they're there. That's a bit like what mixing with people is. It's a bit like those walls. Being able to focus on them. Yeah, it's a bit like those walls - if you're mad you think you can walk through walls, but when you see it physically there, you can't. Do you know what I mean? It's a bit like that really. Unless you're David Copperfield of course. He walks through walls doesn't he. The Great Wall of China. That's a bit weird. Do you reckon he's human? *(laughs)*. .

Let me think. My spiritual experiences are very strange. I was walking along the road one day and this invisible energy thing came up behind me and hit me on the back of the head and it was so real that I thought it had actually happened. I touched my head and my head was still there, so I thought ' well hang on'. That's happened like another time and I sort of fell on the floor but I could also like see myself a couple of steps down the road, walking along. It was a bit weird really. It was like there were two of me, one was killed and the other one wasn't.

The voices went away for a bit and then they came back. They started whispering at first. I'd say to people 'did you say something?' and they'd say no and gradually I realized they were back. At first they were only there when I was stoned and they'd go away when I wasn't. Then gradually they became more permanent again. There was a voice in my head about a year ago that said 'He's got the sight'. Which is how I tend to describe it, my illness, as a sight. The trouble is, all I see with my sight is madness. I see it as this disease that's consuming everything.

Like I said, I'm not Christian or anything like that. I mean, I wouldn't walk with lepers, do you know what I mean? If you're gonna die when you're 32, like Jesus, I suppose it doesn't matter does it? I reckon he could have done his job better hey. I wrote a poem about that called 'The Forsaken Child'. It's about if Jesus really was, like, The Lord, why didn't he stay and lead us instead of dying and leaving us? Why isn't he here for us now? With proof of his power and that. So that we wouldn't be in doubt.

I think my relationship with my parents is a good one. I can only say that because it used to be a bad one. So compared to how it used to be, it's good. I was rebellious. I skived off school. I took drugs. I stole motorbikes. I tortured my mam. They adopted me when I was 6 days old. What it was, my mam that I've got now, well her and her first husband, were trying to have a child. And she kept having miscarriages. They were reading the paper one day and it said 'Wanted. A good home for a baby child'. They had to go to court and make it legal. It's almost apparent though that we're from different families, 'cos, you know, I was like a tearaway and that and all they ever did was work hard, 9 to 5, you know. They didn't swear at other people or nothing, do you know what I mean? They never got into fights or anything. It was like I'm from a completely different neck of the woods. She – me mam - used to say, 'Well nobody else in our family did things like that'. And they didn't. I think she loves me though. As a mother. More than most women would love a child, because I was wanted. I wasn't something that accidentally happened *(pauses)*... It's not even as simple as that really. I was more than wanted. I was went and got *(laughs)*.

I've got two mothers and three fathers. I was going to find about who my blood parents were 'cos that's two of them, but it doesn't matter about that at the moment. My mam doesn't want me to,now, so you know, I'm not gonna upset her anymore than I have already. I'll just have to leave it. Perhaps when she's gone, I'll try and find out if they're still alive. Perhaps they will be, perhaps they won't. I might not even be here. Who knows? I might go before me mam.

My illness has stressed my mam right out over the years. One time they had a bloody riot van out the front of the house. Loads of coppers in the house with riot shields. Theres me stood there with this bloody axe thing. Things like that. There's another time when they came to pick me up to section me, I punched one in the mouth outside and legged it. I was on the run for a month once, with a warrant on me and all sorts of things like that, you know. That's why I say now, I have a good relationship with my parents. I mean when you compare it with that, it's not difficult.

I've got a sister. My second mother's real daughter. She's younger than me though. They said in the hospital, perhaps when you adopted him, it gave you the mothering instinct. That's just daft really. I think it just worked for her that time. My sisters about 14 months younger than me. That's my niece who you saw when you came in. My sister and I put up with one another nowadays. We used to fight all the time when we was kids.

When I was about 20, I met a woman. Purely by accident really. I got deeply involved with her. She was like a hippy, into veganism and all that sort of stuff. At the time I was very confused about my voices. But 'erm, I became very disturbed by the voices in association with this lady. And, the time I was telling you about with the coppers, for example, it was because in my head there was like people raping her all the time and it wasn't just physical rape, it was like mental rape and torture and all this sort of stuff. This carried on for a couple of years.

People kidnapped her and carted her off to places around the world. I was trying to do something about it but in a mad way. Of course it never really happened. Only in my head it happened. It was like I saw her as the earth and everybody wanted to rape her. So she was very important in that aspect and I went completely barmy over her.

She was like a hippy and she lived in this camper van thing and I went there and I broke into her van. When she came home, she threw a barney and told me to leave. So I gave her a kick. I'd never hit her before. It's the only time I ever did hit her. Anyway, she ran off and come back with these couple of people. They were like okay about it.

They just talked to me, you know, and that's all I needed to do really, was just talk to her, to sort things out. But she didn't want to know, she was really stressed out. Around my mental illness, people do get really stressed out because I get really freaky. Do you know what I mean? They head for the hills, I can tell you.

She fucked me up basically. Now I look back on it, it was a learning process for me. My voices went really weird. Some really strange things happened. I got into this really weird mental war thing. All out mental war it was. She sort of kicked it off, well I suppose it weren't really her fault. I met her in a pub. She was a barmaid. I don't have nothing to do with women normally. I was there with my mate. He said to me 'I like that bird', about one of the other barmaids. 'Why don't you pick one of the other ones? It just sort of happened like that. I never had sex with her or nothing. The next day I went down the pub. I took some poems with me and it started there. They were crap poems as well*(laughs)*... women! I don't know.

I've come a long way from there. She helped me in a way, she was like a catalyst, you know, she kicked things off for me. Like being a vegan. She was like a starting gun, you know, at the beginning of a race.

What really made that lass important, was, because before then when I used to talk about my voices with people, they just said 'you're mad, forget it', but she didn't see. One night I had this dream about her and I saw her the next day and she'd dreamt about me too. That got the ball rolling for me, it was like a very specific point. That was why she was more important than she would have otherwise been. I thought that I'd made a sort of connection with her, a sort of psychic connection and that was like a proof that the voices and thoughts were more than just madness. That's how she became more important than she would otherwise have been. I'd bit into it and I wouldn't let go. It just escalated after that, pretty much.

I was practicing with telepathy. Like for instance with my nan. She used to live next door and she used to come over every night. She was deaf and when I was speaking to her, I used to try thinking the words into her head at the same time I'd be speaking to her. She seemed to be able to hear me when I talked, whereas she didn't hear other people. I believe in mind over matter, or telekinesis as they call it. Basically I've got my religion, I've found the tools I need amongst the madness. So I don't need to go on about things like that anymore because I am where I am. In them days I didn't know what was what. That woman, she created a very important milestone that I had to pass through, that's what's so important about her, she was a milestone. Like with the dream and the veganism, and the conflicts I got into about her afterwards. I used to wander mindlessly round the countryside looking for her and she wasn't there *(laughs)*.

I became a vegan because of her and my religion. It's taken me 15 years to develop my religion. It might sound simple, but it's not. I write it down and it's almost like writing a formula. It's like my poetry, it's serious stuff and I can go back to it, and I know where I'm at when I read it.

The voices haven't changed over the years. They're just evil. What's changed is how I relate to them. I mean, I still get ill now and again. I cut my throat. Look (shows scar). Blood was pouring down onto the tarmac outside, on the concrete. And I used to burn myself with a lighter. When I did the burning, I was thinking 'right, I'm going to hell. I got to get used to the pain so that I can fight against it or whatever, and not succumb to it'. But since then.... well I've learnt they just lock you away in hospital if you do things like that. There's no point is there? What do they call it? There's a phrase isn't there? Yeah, there's a phrase that describes it. But anyway, if I'm going to spend the next however many years shut away in some hospital, not allowed to have a lighter, there's not a lot of point in burning myself. That's what I thought afterwards anyway, because I mean, I had blisters over my fingers, my hands and everything.

I cut my throat because I was in a lot of physical pain. You know what the popular image of what the devil looks like. You know, pointed ears, bat wings, tail, horns, that sort of thing. Well, my mental self took on that form. Witches call them abstract bodies. It took on that kind of form. So I was like a devil and lots of my voices were trying to kill it and the pain was really physical. In my head. I could hardly move. There were these other voices. They were supposed to be Hell's Angels. Anyway, they said 'We're going to do that to your whole family', my niece and all that, you know. They said 'if you kill yourself, we'll let 'em off'. So I tried to do it, but I didn't quite get there.

But it's like every time you survive something like that you learn something, like now if the voices said that again, I'd say 'well, fuck you ' because I know they're not true to their word. They didn't kill anybody. I was chatting to a guy the other week and he hears voices now and again. I mean I hear mine every minute of every day, you know. Anyway I was chatting to him and he said his were saying that all of the North West is going to come round and do him over. I said to him 'Yeah, I gets that all the time' and I do. But I mean... *(pauses)* then it doesn't happen. I mean to me, it's like sorting the truth from the lies. Sorting the madness from the reality and all that sort of stuff. I think I'm privileged really. Most people they get this madness and they either become Christians, or they become totally insane because it's so overwhelming. I've been able to sift through it like…. like I might think that the kids I grew up with are going to come round and kick my head in because the voices are telling me so, you know. Well it doesn't happen. And the more it doesn't happen, the less I'm afraid of it. That's what surviving is, you know to become less afraid of something. To come out of the other end of it and still believe in something without believing in Christianity or Islam or some thing organized like that, is a real achievement.

Hospital? I thought I'd been in there about 10 times, but apparently they've got me written down as being in there about 20 odd. I've been in that many times and I can't remember them. I don't know what they've been doing to me. It's not a very nice place really. I don't like hospital. It's terrible in fact. You think, 'OK, I'll go into hospital, I'll have a nice rest' but it ain't like that. There's like an atmosphere in there, you could cut it with a knife, you know. And the nurses are all smiles, saying 'take this you'll feel better.' A typical example is, when I went in once and I'd just stopped smoking cannabis before I went in and I was telling one of the nurses and he said to me, 'Oh I could get you some if you want'. Do you know what I mean? I reported the incident. I mean I didn't report the culprit, but I reported the incident to the people higher up. They asked me who it was and I wouldn't tell them. But stuff like that does go on but no one believes you, because you're mad.

Another time I went in hospital they were trying to change my medication and 'um, they managed to wean me off this stuff and I said 'Right, I'm not gonna take this either'; the *new* stuff. I want to see how I am without it, that I'm OK without it. And I thought I was okay. I wasn't angry with anyone anymore. I wasn't paranoid or anything like that. And then they decided to section me because I wouldn't take any medication and to do that, well I wasn't having it and I said 'I've had enough of this. I'm leaving'. And they put me on - well, there's different types of section orders and the one they put me on was where the nurse on their own has the power to hold me for - I think it's half a day, and then one doctor's got the power to hold me for another day - or is it three days or something like that. By that time I've got to see a doctor, a social worker and I'm not sure what the third person is, then they can section me for 6 months. Anyway that's what they did and in that order. That was because I didn't want to take my medication and they decided I had to. So no, I don't like hospitals.

The medication helps make me happy but to tell you the truth, I don't like taking it. Basically, if I stop taking medication at home, there's nothing they can do about it so long as I don't get ill. My mam gets really upset if I don't take it though, so I take it for her really. But for the last couple of days I've been cutting one of the tablets into 4 and just been having 3 bits of it. So I've cut out 25 mg of it basically. I haven't told my mam though. She'd go potty if she knew. Even with that small difference, I feel better in myself you know. I'm not ravenously hungry like I normally am. So it's interesting really. I'm trying to get down to 100mg. I've been down to 100 a couple of times and then I stopped it altogether and you get like fever and diarrhoea and all that because it's so addictive. It's not something you can just stop taking easily because you get all these withdrawal effects. Also another thing that happened was that I couldn't sleep. Two weeks solid I didn't get hardly any sleep. Just couldn't sleep. I had fever, I had diarrhoea. I couldn't eat. I was vomiting. That was just because I stopped taking the medication. And you say to the doctor, 'Look at me. Look. Look, I'm like this. This isn't right.' And they say 'Oh, start taking the medication again and you'll be alright'. Do you know what I mean? It's not right.

Basically I've gotta take it in my own hands. I used to smoke pot all the time, you know, I was addicted to that. Now I'm vegan and all that, I don't want to take any kind of drug. It's just a lifestyle thing really. I don't really want the medication. I mean if I was into drugs I might but I'm not anymore. Clozaril...the good thing about Clozaril is it hasn't got as many side effects as the other psychiatric medicines, and it does make you feel happy. It puts a smile on your face. You think maybe the world isn't so bad after all. And if it is, I don't care *(laughs)* .... Do you know what I mean? That's about it really. That's the good side to the Clozaril. So if you're into medication or drugs, get a bit of Clozaril. The trouble is it messes your blood up. You have to keep having blood tests. So it's not the sort of thing some druggies are gonna get into.

I like to talk about my schizophrenia. Like I say, it's spiritual for me. It incorporates my religious beliefs as well, my lifestyle you know. I talk about it just to try and make them think. To think to themselves 'what am I doing?'. I just want them to think really. I do want to talk about what's important. Love and peace and all that man.

I mean I see the medical profession as being there to support me in times of weakness and all that. So I do like to talk to people involved in the profession about my voices and stuff. Whereas people outside it can be difficult, you know. What is it they say, you should never talk about? What is it? Sex, religion or politics? Is that the three of them? Yeah, well I think mental illness is among them in a way. It's something that isn't talked about.

It's like with me mam, you know. It's how I get on with her. I don't talk to her about how I'm feeling or anything. I can't. And it's kind of better that way. We just sort of live round each other, you know. I make her cups of tea you know. She calls me in the morning to get up. That's pretty much it. We've had forty odd years of living together. Bit like a man and wife.

I think people are aware of mental illness and I think they just see you as being like a second class type of person. People think that mental illness is something you should keep to yourself, do you know what I mean? Rather than go round telling people. Yeah, that's what I reckon. Even the people at the drop-in, where I go, even there. You can't talk to the clients about your illness, not unless they're well enough to take on board what you're saying. Because, you know, quite often people are just too ill to listen. That's why the staff are needed. Like I say, Social Workers and all that. They say to me, who would you get in touch with if you were ill? I seem to be the only person who goes to the drop-in that says 'The Samaritans', because they're always there, you know, 24 hours a day. You can have a cup of tea and all that because they've got an office down town that's open now and again. I always say 'The Samaritans'. The rest of the people that there, the rest of the clients, they think The Samaritans are crap, but I don't think so at all. I think as a last ditch, they're really good, you know. Because I mean, I had a meeting the other day with my CPN and he said you know 'Who would you contact in an emergency?', 'What services?'. Because like, my CPN is only there a couple of days a week, so I can't always call him. The hospitals are only open during the day. So, at the end of the day, I'll say The Samaritans because they're there all the time.

They've said to me recently I might be able to help other people that are ill cope with the illness. My psychiatrist said, apparently there's some kind of work going on, where people who have been or who are mentally ill, but who've learnt to cope with it can go along to the other people who are mentally ill and try and sort them out. But it's a bit difficult really you can't force things on people, you know, I've learnt that through my religion. I'll have to give it a go and see how it works. Maybe I've found a niche in society where I slot in.

What's helped me? Well, like I say, I've found this religion thing. I practice that and it's like a magical medicine. I say a prayer. To who? Well, it's a bit difficult. Some people would say God. I'm not sure about this big bang thing though. I think perhaps there are a lot of Gods and they made a lot of stars. I prefer to call it the host. You know, we live in a garden that is provided for us by the host. But I'll say a prayer. In a way, it is God I'm speaking to I suppose.

What else do I do? I was going to say something earlier about this physical health thing but I got sidetracked. It's important. That's why I stopped smoking and drinking. Being physically healthy is important. Healthy body, healthy mind type thing. If you've got a healthy body it makes you feel good. Do you know what I mean? If you look a million dollars in your birthday suit and you're walking down the street with some snazzy outfit on, it's gonna make you feel good as well, you know. Hey, who's the man, you know? This is why I want to give my medication up. It does mess you up physically. It's like being a drunkard, you know, or someone who's stoned all the time, it messes with your body. I don't know if you've seen people who smoke hash all the time, Cannabis or whatever. But they're like really skinny. Well with my medication it works the other way. I've got my dumb bells, I do them for 3-4 hours a day, every day. And I walk, well I cheat. I take a long time over it. Really, I should do it a lot quicker, but I don't and I just have big breaks in between like, you know. As long as I do about 5 miles a day or so, I'm happy.

Like I say, I cut that little corner off my tablet, so now I'm not so ravenous. I'm not eating like a pig now, like I would eat a couple of days ago. It's all physical. It's not so much just looking good. If you're healthy, then you feel good. I mean, I think there's natural medicines. It's like coffee, you know. I mean medication can make you constipated. So I started drinking coffee again. I hadn't drunk coffee for ages until recently. I started drinking coffee again and I'm on the loo all the time. But, I mean I'd rather do that because I mean, if you're constipated it's horrible. I don't know if you've ever been like that? Your stomach feels bloated and you don't want to move and it's all uncomfortable and everything. Yeah, so I mean like I say, it makes you happy being healthy. So I mean, it's just a case of finding what works for you really, if you want to feel happy. If you want to get stoned, smoke cannabis. But I don't want to get stoned anymore. I'm into this healthy buzz. I think it's incredible. If you go round for 15 years stoned out of your mind and you have hospital medication and all that, when you start stopping all that, you realize how powerful life really is. You feel things. Like straight life, you know. The adrenalin, the sexual emotions and 'um, stuff like laughing at jokes. It's incredible, the power of the emotions, because they get really subdued on drugs and medication. It's like a commonly asked question is er, 'does the medication affect your sex life?' You know, and um it does subdue the emotions involved. It's quite surprising really, how powerful these emotions really are.

I do think my religion is all tied in with my psychosis. I think it's the other side to the madness. I call it the father of all religions. It's written in the stars. I think I'm very lucky to have found it. Obviously I've looked very hard for it. To me personally, my religion means the difference for me between heaven and hell.

If you want to know more about the actual schizophrenia itself, well, take the voices for example. The voices try to be like, for example, they try to be, like angels and demons and God and the devil and spacemen and computers and animals and planets, ghosts and witches, policemen, Hell's Angels, Christian church people and Muslims. You name it, they'll try to be it. They try to be Jupiter and it's moons and the sun. I think mine's a full blown version. The thing is, see, that religion of mine that I've uncovered, well you read the Bible and the Bible condemns the religion that I've got - so the way the voices work is, well they're presenting an alternative view point, there's two sides to the argument. Some of the voices support my religion and then there's those that don't. The two sides are, well, if the Christian God rules the earth that means that I'm satanic, but because I know my religion really is a good one, then that means the Bible's got to be satanic, and my voices are always arguing about that. They play on it.

One of my voices said recently 'Oh, we've got a new player', meaning me when I tried to reason with them. As if it's a game. But it's not a game really. They come from the telly sometimes. They use the telly to time travel *(laughs)*. That's a bit weird, that is. But what it, what it basically is, is that the voices are fighting and it's got to be played out, you know, and I have to win because otherwise I lose my mind to it and I go mentally insane or the whole world dies or something like that. And it's like it's a fight you know in my head. That's what it's like really.

Sometimes the voices turn into maggots inside my brain, eating my brain. I said a prayer to my voices a long time ago. I said 'Look there's hell going on in my head. Please try and help me.' I get the Pope in my head a lot. He's trying to convert me. One of the common angles my voices take is that I'm such a fucking wimp that even the people of my religion wouldn't want me.

Yeah, welcome to the Land of Craigy. Keep out.

Bill

Bill responded to an advert I put out requesting volunteers to be interviewed. He spoke candidly and with ease about his life and mental health problems with little need for coaxing from me. He lives with his partner and is currently looking for employment.

I had a messed up childhood from day one. My mum left home when I was two and a half because she couldn't take the beatings any more off my dad. My dad then turned his attention to his kids *(laughs)* and being the youngest, I received more than my share of it. Including my dad taking me out doing burglaries and such at the age of seven years old onwards *(laughs)*. I got involved in drinking at around the same age as well.

I was brought up in a little village in the middle of no-where... *(laughs)* You know, there was three main names in the village sought of thing, and I was in one of them brackets. So it was just one of them things. I got moved around a lot. I think the longest I stayed in any one place was about 10 months.

This was in Wales, South Wales. And, well, I did various stints with my grandparents, my dad and various girlfriends. My Auntie and Uncle. The local kids home. I can remember going back and forwards and seeing child psychologists and what not, in the local health centre. And I can remember going to see them as early like 5-6 years old, because the adults thought I was a problem *(laughs)*. After that I kind of graduated along the criminal path. Being introduced to it at such an early age, it was inevitable that I was going to be getting involved with people who were doing much more than what I was. By the time I got to thirteen and I got in touch with my mum, I was already in my second comprehensive school, having been kicked out of the first.

There was a disagreement with another school down the road and I was one of the ringleaders. We organised a large group of us to go down there for a major ruck. And I got suspended for a fortnight for that one. That was 'cos I kicked a brace down a guys throat in a fight. And I got back and within a week of getting back; someone wholloped me and spun me round and the first thing I saw was the fire extinguisher. So I picked it up and hit him in the face a few times with the bottom of it, and they expelled me *(nervous laugh)*. I just kind of lost it. You know what I mean? I'd had enough. *(laughs)* It was a case of I'd taken abuse for years off my dad and there was just - there's only so much that anybody's gonna take before they think, well okay, enough's enough now *(laughs)*.

Anyway at thirteen, I managed to get in touch with my mum. She lives up this way and I'd had no contact with her at all up until then. I'd been asking about her from the moment I could speak and realised that she wasn't about. You know what I mean? I wanted to see her. And it took eleven years for my grandparents to get the address that they had for her father out of the sideboard.

They'd had it in the sideboard all along, but they just weren't willing to get it out. And then they wrote the letter off to her. My mum only got it because she was clearing out her dad's house. He'd passed away. If it had been left another week or two, she would never of got it and I'd never of had contact with her. But I came up here and I got introduced to drugs *(laughs)*. I turned up at my mum and step dad's house and they were dealing. So that was my introduction. Yep. They were selling hash from the house, so I got introduced to that first of all. I was already in a situation where I knew I could earn a lot of money doing the crime thing. And, well, I kinda snowballed from hash and got involved with various other things.

I don't have anything to do with any of my brothers and sisters now. As I said I'm the youngest of six. My eldest brother, Adam, he's only been out of Dartmoor a couple of years. He did a seven year stretch out of a twelve year sentence. And he's only been out a couple of years and he's in South Wales and I'm up here, so that's that. My two other brothers, there's Kieran and Daniel. Kieran's a regimental Sergeant Major in the army. Well if you pardon my French, I think he's a complete prick *(laughs)*. Then there's my brother Daniel, he's an officer on a nuclear submarine. Because he's an officer, he believes he is better than the rest of us. As far as I'm concerned, he's an even bigger prick *(laughs)*. As for my sisters, well, I don't have anything to do with them either. If they have a problem then they will get in touch with me *(laughs)*. It's about the only time they will, if they need me for something. Other than that I don't have anything to do with them. I have no contact with my Welsh side of the family.

My eldest brother, he copped a lot of the flack before I did. It was a case of by the time my dad looked and realised how big my oldest brother was getting, he looked around and the others were getting a bit large as well. I'm the smallest out of us all and *(laughs)* well, I copped it then, sort of like. Yeah, it was difficult. I can remember my dad's way of solving disagreements very well. It was a pair of boxing gloves each and 'step out into the backyard' job. Whoever's standing at the end of it is the one who is in the right. It didn't matter whether it was brother arguing against brother, sister against sister, or brother against sister. You got given a pair of gloves each and sent out the back *(laughs)*. I mean it was just the way we were brought up *(laughs)*. I can remember going to school with bruises all over me, where he had battered me with the buckle end of the belt. I'd answered him back. It was a really strict family unit, you know what I mean? Held together with force.

My grandparents did the majority of the upbringing for most of us. My grandfather was one of them people well, he only ever raised his hand to me once and I'd already left home by that time. My gran stopped him and told him not to. In all honesty, I would of hurt him. I was doing all sorts of things and into everything at the time. I wasn't in my right mind at all. I would of hurt him. But he never raised a hand to any of us before that, my grampy. All he had to do was raise his voice and we would jump and do what he said *(laughs)*. My gran, well, she treated me as a little kid until the day I left. I mean I left home at fifteen and up until the time I left, my gran was cutting the Mars Bar up into bite-sized pieces and putting them on a saucer for me. So that I wouldn't have to bite the Mars Bar *(laughs)*. Silly things like that, she, she was just like a really overbearing mother figure sort of thing. But yeah, I have happy memories of my grandparents. You know, I do have pissed off memories about them as well. But they always treated us fair.

They didn't know my dad was taking me out doing burglaries and what not. I knew better than to try and tell them. I already tried telling somebody, one of the school teachers I think, or assistant in the class or something like that. I'd already tried telling one of them about my dad giving me beatings. But unfortunately it was a really small area, everybody knows everybody *(laughs)* so I got told not to tell lies. Then somebody told my dad that I'd been telling lies about him beating me. So I got beaten for that*(laughs)*. I couldn't win, you know what I mean? I learnt it was best not to say anything. I still haven't told my grandmother. She's the only one left now my grampy's gone. I haven't told her because it'd break her heart. To know that her son was taking out her grandson to do things like that, you know what I mean? It would break her heart and I can't do that to her. She's responsible for a lot of my common sense *(laughs)*. I mean there's times where... I mean... I've sat in police interviews and lied white is black and had them persuaded that it is by the end of the interview. I could never tell a lie to my gran *(laughs)*. She knows. She just knows. The minute I start telling one, she knows *(laughs)*. But, er... they were great people. They used to take us away quite regularly. They had a caravan, a big old converted ambulance. They used to take us off for the weekend on it. We'd come home on a Friday from school and it would all be packed up, you know what I mean? It wouldn't be a case of 'right go get your clothes'. They'd already be in there as well *(laughs)*. I'd turn up at home from school in school uniform. My gran would have my clothes laid out on the bed for me to change into. She was that sort of person. She was a really nice woman *(laughs)*. But she, well, none of us could stand up to my dad. (short laugh). It's really unfortunate.

It might have something to do with the fact that he's an evil little shit *(laughs)*. My dad got to the semi-finals in the Welsh Amateur Heavy Weight Boxing Championships when he was four years younger than I am now. He can handle himself. He's worked as a professional bouncer at the rugby club in our village, you know what I mean? And the rugby players don't fuck with my dad *(laughs)*. He's in his late fifties now and they still won't. So, he's, you know, he's a handful. And it's one of them things, he can make life really difficult *(laughs)*. He's like, well, he's well known.

Prime example being a few years back. I'd got a flat back in my home area. I'd been gone for about eight, nine years. But my dad found out I was there and turned up on the flat doorstep and said 'You have one week. I'll give you one week. If you're not gone by the end of that week, if I don't come and move you, I know plenty of people who'll come and do it for me' *(laughs)*. So I had to move out. It had taken me about six years to get a proper housing association council flat. And I had to give it up. I had no choice. *(laughs)*

Anyway like I said I was thirteen when I came up here. My mum and step-dad were dealing and I got involved with that. I stayed up here for a little while. My mum and step-dad taking me back and forth to the children's psychiatric unit. And I don't know how to explain it...

193

(pauses) it's weird but me and my mum were a hell of a lot alike for people who ain't been around each other that much. So like, it was strange being with her, but it wasn't that difficult. It seemed fairly easy. Also my step dad never hit me either in the time I was up here. God knows he had enough reason to on occasions *(laughs)*. But yeah, I was going back and forwards to the psychiatric unit thing up here.

I wasn't quite what you would call a normal young teenager. I mean, I could match my step-dad pint for pint *(laughs)* I mean, he's an ex-Hell's Angel *(laughs)*. He can drink. At thirteen I used to match him pint for pint. I was coming out with things I shouldn't have been coming out with. I was getting involved in rucks for virtually no reason whatsoever. I just seemed to have an extremely violent streak I suppose. They took me back and forwards to this place and then this guy said 'Well, if he's no better next visit, I'd like to keep him in for a couple of days'. My mum gave me the note to take to school and I didn't know the doctor had said this and I read it and I thought 'Sod that' and instead of going to school I just carried on cycling. The police picked me up eventually and took me back home, to my mum's. And they put me straight into a secure kids home. Bars on the windows there *(laughs)*. Thirteen I was, coming up fourteen.

I was only there for about a month before my grampy came up and took me out. My mum had phoned my grampy in Wales to tell him that I was in there and the following morning he turns up. He walked in and told them that he was taking me. When they said 'You can't, his mum has signed him in' he said 'I don't give a fuck. I'm his legal court appointed guardian. I haven't signed any paper work. You either give him to me now or I'll come back with a court order saying you have to'. So they let me go *(laughs)*. I went straight back down to Wales then. I didn't even get a chance to go and say goodbye to my mum. My grampy weren't even willing to drive me round there so I could say goodbye and whatnot. *(laughs)* I went back down to Wales and got back into the criminal thing again. Using various different drugs now as well.

While I was with my mum I was smoked quite a bit of hash and only had other stuff now and again. When I got back to Wales and started crooking again, I had all this extra money. There was all this different stuff on the scene and when people realised I was smoking dope, they weren't so worried about showing me other things, and I kind of sunk myself into it really. I think that's where a lot of my illness came from. I used to do large amounts of pure amphetamine. I got in trouble a few times with the police. I ended up on a supervision order at fifteen.

I was mainly doing shop burglaries, house burglaries and warehouses, stuff like that. I weren't doing armed robbery at that point *(laughs)*. That came a year or two later *(laughs)*. But I did get involved quite deeply. Like most people, I started off doing little things and ended up getting deeper and deeper. I actually came up here to retire *(laughs)*. I mean, it was getting scary. I was involved with a lot of dangerous people and it was getting scary. Know what I mean?

I was off my face near enough all the time. I'd wake up in the morning and I'd be having my speed. I'd have a gram ready to put in the syringe for myself and I'd whack that. I'd have three spliffs, half a bottle of Vodka. Then I'd do it all over again and then I'd get out of bed, get dressed *(laughs)*. I'd get off my face from the moment I woke up.

It was the only way I could get by at that point. I ended up committing various different crimes. I got a nine month sentence in Swansea prison in the Young Offenders part. I'd done four months on remand. I thought I only had two weeks to go but I'd lost all my remission. Because of charges I'd had before I'd been sentenced. So when I got my sentence, it took all my remission. The same happened a second time. I didn't lose it all straight off. I lost a chunk of it and just thought then 'oh sod it' *(laughs)*. They can't give me any extra time, you know what I mean? Then I did four months on remand. I got given a choice. The judge did basically give me a choice. It was a case of go to the Ley Community[15] on twelve months conditional residency with a probation order, or I could have an eight year custodial sentence. They were finally beginning to have enough by now. I was up in the top five of the ones in the area that they wanted to bang up and get off the scene *(laughs)*. So I took the Ley *(laughs)*. Yes, I took the Ley Community and it was while I was there that I got diagnosed.

I did ten months out of a twelve month period at the Ley. And I think, within a month of getting there, the doctor that they used at the time actually diagnosed me and had me on a dead ball injection.

Schizophrenia was the immediate diagnosis. Then it was paranoid schizophrenia with psychotic tendencies. That is because when I get ill, I see things. Retreat into my own little space sort of thing. Which, well, that's just the nature of it.

I'd gone into the Ley Community and they don't give you anything to help you come off drugs. You come off cold turkey and you still have to be part of the community, do you know what I mean? I'd kind of had these things going on in my mind for a while anyway before I went in. I'd been

---

[15] The Ley Community is a drug and alcohol rehabilitation centre

hearing people saying something to me and then there'd be nobody there. I knew that there was something a bit dodgy but I kind of put it down to the drugs *(laughs)*. When I was coming off in that first month, coming off the cold turkey bit, I kind of put a lot of what was going through my head down to the detox and what not. The actual coming off thing.

It wasn't until a month or so into the Ley that I started thinking, well hang on a minute, I really shouldn't be having these, that it couldn't be down to the drugs or the detox. Then the diagnosis came and they declared me unsuitable for work *(laughs)*.

Anyway I was there for ten months and I know it a terrible thing to say, but there's many a time I wished I picked the eight years. Rather than being in the Ley Community. It did give me some guidelines, hints on how to deal with my addictions. But I'd taken what I'd thought was the easy option in court. Given a choice between eight years and twelve months, what is any person going to choose? And, well now, I'd rather have been in prison.I wasn't ready to do it. I wasn't going to get the most out of it at the time. I was going there because it's the easier of two options available.

You'd have sessions where you had a confrontational style group. I usually ended up on a punishment contract after those. I'm... not very good with lots of people giving me grief. If somebody has a problem with me and then says 'Look Bill, I have a problem with you because you do this, can you work something out?', then I'll try and work something out with them and I'll apologise if it's out of order. You know what I mean? But if I've got one person starting to have a pop at me, and then I've got three or four other people jumping in because they always work the groups out so as to air as many grievances as possible. So you might be sat there with half a dozen people screaming at you. Then I'd shout back at 'em and then you've got the entire group bombing you sort of thing. Giving you verbal abuse and whatnot. And I just couldn't cope with it. I used to lose my rag. I'd end up on punishment duty near enough every time *(laughs)*. I just can't cope with that sort of thing.

There were loads of rules and regulations. Everybody in there had to take part in the running of the community. All you had was a basic structure of staff at the top and they were all ex-addicts who had been through the programme themselves. So, like it wasn't as if it was easy to get anything by them *(laughs)*. I did the ten months, then I came out. I had to go and see probation and the probations officer said 'Ok, I won't breach you, you've lasted longer than most people that get sent there by the courts' *(laughs)*. Anyhow I left and ended up going to a hostel and then I went back down to Cardiff. Back down to Wales.

I'd been diagnosed by this time and I was on medication. I was hearing voices. I hear voices 24/7. They never go away, not even with medication. They just quieten. They become easier to cope with. I can't actually pinpoint specific time that they started. They were just there. They seem to have been there for an awfully long time. I know it sounds strange but by the time I realised that they were there, they'd been there for a hell of a long time *(laughs)*. It was one of them situations of, well, I can't honestly couldn't say when it started. You know, I was diagnosed at eighteen and a half but I'd been seeing psychologists and psychiatrists since I was like five or six years old *(laughs)*.

I couldn't say I was hearing voices at that point in time because I can't remember that I was, but er... I was obviously, there was obviously something wrong with me 'cos every adult that I went to stay with in the family ended up taking me to see a psychologist or psychiatrist. There must have been something.

I'm thirty-one. So it's been roughly thirteen years since I was diagnosed. I've been on medication constantly since then. I'm on a new-ish drug now. It's not too bad. I find that it can make me drowsy and I can have difficulty being able to get on with things. So quite often if I've got things I need to do throughout the day, I won't take my morning tablet. Not until I've finished with what I've had to do in the day, which can quite often end up with me having to do two tablets in the space of like an hour and a half, when you're not supposed to really. But I don't have much option. If I take it first thing, I want to go back to bed *(laughs)*. It's not that I'm lazy, just that it messes you up. It's worse than a lot of the drugs that they class as illegal *(laughs)*. You know what I mean? I smoke pot on a regular basis too. I find that it is more helpful to me than a lot of medication that the doctors supply.

I get stressed out quite regularly. I can get really - like I want to hit things, hit my own head and things at times. I can get really frustrated. I kind of figure it's a lot better for me to sit down and smoke a reefer than to sit down and take 30-40 ml of valium, drink two or three cups of coffee and smoke half a dozen fags while I'm waiting for the valium to kick in. I think that smoking a reefer is a lot better for me and causing a lot less damage to my body.

It calms me down. Calms my mind and whatnot. I use it medically. It is a case of ... I can't function properly unless I've had a smoke sort of thing. I'm too stressed out about going outdoors and everything, you know what I mean? So it's a case of, well, I have to get by . I mean, I hate going out and being around crowds of people. I have to calm myself down before I can even go and do shopping or anything. At least I'm still capable of doing stuff if all I've had is a reefer. If I've had to take 30-40 ml of valium I'm not going to be any good wandering around the supermarket *(laughs)*. It's that simple. I need something to keep me going. To keep me calm, but I can still do things. Unfortunately a lot of the medication the doctors give you, it will calm you down alright, but you just don't want to move after you have taken it *(laughs)*. Well, this works for me, it doesn't necessarily mean it will work for anyone, but it does for me.

It doesn't help with the voices when I smoke. I mean I don't notice any difference with the voices. I get my good days, I get my bad days whatever. It doesn't seem to make a great deal of difference whether I've been smoking or not. Some days I get up and I can hardly hear them at all. Other days I'll get up they're so loud they're blocking things out that are actually real, you know what I mean? It's not nice.

They're not pleasant. I've got two main ones that are there constantly. There's 'er, a little girl's voice and she's constantly telling me how she is being mentally, sexually and physically abused by this man where they are. Telling that she needs me to go there to fight the man to stop him from doing it. That the only way I can get there is to kill myself to get to where they are. Now, when it's quiet I can cope, but when that's really loud it starts to get a bit insistent and whatnot. The other one is, is the actual bloke who's abusing her. He's really abusive towards me and threatening. Goading me into taking him on sort of thing. And there have been times when it's got to the stage where I thought to myself, 'Right ok, I'm coming to get you now.' I've ended up taking overdoses and attempted to hang myself and...do you know what I mean? There have been occasions when I've done that, twenty-odd at last count. It gets that bad. There are times where I just think to myself, 'ok, that's what I've got to do then I'm going to do it'. And when I do attempt to kill myself they're not half-baked attempts either. I mean, I've taken boxes of major tranquillisers. I've taken - the most I've taken I think was I took three boxes of Chlopromazine tablets. I woke up three days later. In my own bed. *(laughs)* Just woke up three days later. Couldn't move for a day afterwards but it didn't kill me. That's just one attempt, so it can get quite bad with the voices. Especially if there's nothing to do, because then you tend to focus more on them, which is even worse*(pauses)*... There doesn't seem to be a great deal of assistance for anybody with it either.

Anyway after The Ley I went back to Cardiff and there I got back into the crime scene straight away. It's one of the only things I knew how to do. Seeing I wasn't allowed to work legally anyway *(laughs)*. Because I was medically unfit. It seemed like a reasonably good thing to do, to get back into. By this time I was already higher up the scale, sort of thing. I was already, I had already done robberies. Armed robberies. I'd shot at the police car chasing us and all these various different things, you know what I mean. So I'd gone like up a notch in people's estimation, sort of thing, in those circles. I got involved in that and stayed involved in it until I came up to Oxford *(laughs)*.

Well, I suppose one way of looking at me would be to say that I was a cleaner at one point. If there was a weapon that needed to be got rid of I was your man *(laughs)*. If there were other, more bulky items that needed got rid of, then I was also your man for that too *(laughs)*.

Whatever. Whatever was needed, I'd do it. I've burned out buildings so there is no evidence. I've burned out cars so there is no evidence. I've dismantled guns to distribute them over several different counties *(laughs)*. You know what I mean? Various other different bits and pieces I've dismantled and spread out. Did debt collecting. I was not so much, I didn't so much have a reputation as a hard man - which might sound a bit funny considering what I used to do - but I definitely had the reputation of being willing to go that one step further than most people would. Like I say it wasn't that I was hard, you know, but if I took on a job and I said I was going to do it, it got done whatever *(laughs)*. So like, I had that reputation. I could handle myself if necessary. Obviously I'd rather not have to. If I'm going to have to hurt someone, my motto was to hit them with something like an iron bar, an implement of some sort. What's the point of damaging yourself?(*laughs*) I constantly had admissions into hospital through that period.

I had a few relationships while I was down there. I've actually got five kids of my own. By four different mothers. I mean I had a few relationships but the one I'm in now is the longest one I've ever had. I've been with this woman for just over two and a half years, so it's serious. And, I don't do any crime anymore.

The others, well, I was a crook and I was involved with other crooks. We had lots of money and there was always women hanging about. Relationships don't fair well in that sort of thing *(laughs)*. It is a typical thing of Friday night with the missus, Saturday night with the girlfriend *(laughs)*. You know what I mean? That was that sort of situation I was in and people I mixed with.

There was one woman I got really involved with and I've realised now that I fucked that relationship up myself. I was dishonest. She thought I was no longer using drugs and I was. I was still injecting. She found out and then she discovered some of the people that I was knocking around with were too and realised what sort of people they were. She wanted out so she just walked away. That's the only one that pisses me off when I think about it(*laughs*). But then I come up here and I don't do it no more *(laughs)*. I've had enough.

I'd been doing the drugs from thirteen onwards and I'm still using cannabis on a daily basis. And the crime well, from seven up until - just a sec, I've been up here four years, four and a half years, something like that – and it was right up until I came here.

There were times when I would go in (to hospital) for a couple of weeks just to be in an environment where I could get myself together. Then there were times when I was sectioned for six months at a time. It didn't always help *(laughs)*. Sometimes I was in there on a six month section feeling perfectly well had and there'd be visitors coming into the ward and mistaking me for staff *(laughs)*. And they still wouldn't allow me to go off the ward. I mean that didn't help at all. I suppose sometimes it helped. Other times it was a complete waste of time. Some of the staff in there shouldn't be in the positions they're in. They're not suitable for the job.

What do I mean? Some of them don't have the right temperament. They don't take time to actually be with the patient. Prime example being, when my missus was admitted last year we were going through the process of moving. I was having to arrange all the moving, everything. She's in hospital on a section and I'm really stressed out and there's this nurse sat on the steps at the hospital looking at us, laughing at us cause we're arguing. He stopped laughing when I turned round and told him what I thought of him. But, in that sort of environment, that's not the right attitude for someone in that job to take. Do you know what I mean? *(laughs)*. And they just don't take any time. They'd rather have a sit down and a cup of coffee a lot of the time rather than spend five minutes finding out what's wrong with somebody. They always wait until it blows up before they do anything. Some of them just shouldn't be there.

I moved here because I wanted to retire. It was that simple. In my last month in Cardiff I had three different people pull guns on me. It was getting too much *(laughs)*. It was time to leave. The first one I knew, and I knew didn't have the bottle, so I screamed and ran at him and he ran away. The second one, he did have the bottle, I knew him too, so I ducked and ran away. And the third time, this guy pulled a gun and I didn't know him and before I had a chance to make my mind up, he blew the wind shield out of the car next to me. Missed me by a tiny bit. I ran. And I filled my shorts as I ran. I don't care how brave a man is, if you've got somebody shooting at you, that is getting scary. I decided at that point it was time to get out. That time I'd had enough.*(laughs)*.

I see my mum regularly now, but that's only been in the past few months. My dad, I've had no contact with since I was sixteen. Well there was this one time I told you about, when I'd managed to get a flat in my home area and he put the kybosh on that, so I ended up coming up here. I saw my, well, I haven't seen my gran for, its got to be eight, nine years now. It's been a while. My dad won't let her. My dad won't allow it.

It was difficult up here at first. Even though I could of got the housing through the council, I actually went out of my way to find something myself, with a private landlord. That didn't last very long. I don't take very well to bullying and the letting agents were bullies. I weren't having it, and I told them as much.

They started turning up all threatening at the door. I started answering the door with a twelve inch kitchen knife. You know they were just turning up being mouthy and being verbally abusive, trying to get me to cow down sort of thing. This was just the way they acted towards their tenants, sort of thing, because they thought they could get away with it. But they weren't going to do that with me. I started answering the door with a twelve inch kitchen knife and they didn't like that at all *(laughs)*. Then I ended up moving from there and it took me a while, but now I'm with my missus and her daughter and we've got a little house together.

We met through a mutual friend, well at the time he was a mutual friend but we've since had a falling out. He caused a lot of problems for me and the missus. I think mainly because he was hoping to get in there. He'd known her for years and he introduced me to her and within a month or two *(laughs)*, we were an item. So that pissed him off a bit because he'd introduced us and we really hit it off. We've got a really good relationship. I mean, I'm no longer using hard drugs whatsoever. I haven't done since I've been with her, for over two and a half years now. Also I used to drink a hell of a lot. These days I have bottles of Stella and I tend to have about two or three of them in the evening. It's not a major problem anymore. I've actually started putting weight on. There was a time when I was eight stone. Now I'm something like thirteen *(laughs)*. It's a good relationship. I'm happy.

I think the world of her daughter and I hope her daughter thinks the world of me as well. She's seven. She's really nice. She comes up to my mums and my step-dads with me, and she calls them nanny and grampy *(laughs)*. Yes, it's nice. It's taken me a hell of a long time to be able to get to a situation where I'm on an even keel. I'm still trying to get assistance. Trying to get into a mental health day centre here and trying to get a CPN or some kind of psychiatric worker, because at the moment all I've got is my psychiatrist and GP. I have no other support. It's a bit like, I need a... I need somebody I can contact if I've got a problem, who can help me sort things out. I can't go to a GP with lots of problems. It's really difficult, but I've been knocked back every time I've applied for help.

I haven't got a clue why. Before I came up here, when I was in Cardiff, I had two CPNs, psychiatric social worker, a support worker, and I had to see my GP every week and my psychiatrist every week. But I come up here and I see my psychiatrist once in a blue moon. I see my GP when I need some more tablets *(laughs)*. That's it. I don't have anything else. I think it's really diabolical. I have this long term illness and if they were to look at my files they would see that I have this long term illness and how it has helped having support in the past. It's not a case of, you know, wanting them to be around to do everything for me, but if I'm starting to get unwell, surely it has got to be better for me to be able to find someone out who can help actually stop it when I'm starting, rather than letting it escalate into some big blow up thing. You know what I mean? Then I'll end up banged up on the ward then for months on end, do you know what I mean?... *(laughs)*. It would be much easier to have them step in at the beginning, but they don't seem to accept that. You do get people out there who want the help and can't get it and people who don't want the help and it's being heaped on them. It's unfortunate. *(laughs)*

My missus has mental health issues as well and I support her as well. It can be difficult at times. I mean, touch wood neither of us have well, we've not been ill together. Thankfully that hasn't happened. But er... there are times when it gets really difficult.

As I say I've had various suicide attempts. I start getting paranoid at people who are out to get me. If I have to go out in that sort of situation, I will always carry some kind of weapon. (short laugh). It is, it's my way of thinking, well right, I know they're out to get me so if they come after me then I'm going to have something with me so that I can do some damage back. *(laughs)*. That's when it gets dangerous, when it gets to *that* stage because if I'm that paranoid then it's not much of a big step to think, ah there's the person that wants me, I'm going to have him before he has a chance. You know what I mean? It's not that big a step. I have hurt people in the past.

A lot of the triggers are down to stress. If I'm getting stressed out about different things. I mean, you don't need a big thing to get stressed over. You can have half a dozen little things which will more than do the job. *(laughs)*. But I'll get stressed out and I'll start getting snappy and what not, unless I take time out and actually try to get my head round it and try and sort things out in my own mind. It can get a bit dodgy at that point *(laughs)*. It's not the best thing in the world.

I saw my eldest daughter and my twin boys about five or six years ago at Christmas. When I knocked on the front door they answered and asked who I was. I told them I was their father and they said 'You can't be, daddy's in the house' *(laughs)*. I haven't been back since.

I know they're looked after. They're taken care of. Nobody's going to bother them. It would not be a wise decision. They have very large uncles roaming around my home village. My eldest brother's back in the area, so I know they're going to be well looked after. I know no-ones going to be able to take liberties with them *(laughs)*. But I haven't had anything to do with them at all, so I can't really go stamping in now and disrupting things, you know what I mean? They've got their families.

I did try to have contact with my youngest at one point, just after she was born. I didn't know that this woman had had a child by me because I had split up with her by then and she hadn't told me. But I'd been told by people that she'd had my kid. So I spots her when I'd just picked up a load of hash and speed and whatnot from where I used to go in Cardiff. I was in hospital at the time actually but I'd been let out for the afternoon.*(laughs)* I spotted her pushing the pram and I had a huge wedge of cash on me because I'd been to cash in my book but until that day I'd been confined to the ward up so I'd had nothing to spend it on. I ran over to give her some money to buy something for the baby and I got like ten foot from her, she shouted at me 'Fuck off, don't come any closer. Come any closer I'm shouting for the police'. Considering I had about half an ounce of speed and an ounce of pot on me, plus a wedge of cash, I didn't want to get lifted by the old bill, so I walked off and that was as close as I got to my youngest (short laugh). The other one I've had absolutely nothing to do with. So (long pause)... I realise it's not what I should have done, but then again, their mothers didn't want me involved either.

Looking back on it, remembering all of the shit I was up to at the time and the people I was hanging round with, the people who had disagreements with me and the types of retaliations they could pull, I can fully understand why they didn't want me involved when the kids were born. *(laughs)* My job wasn't nice. Petrol bombs were not unusual. At one point there was a landlord who was refusing to pay his membership money. I think that was the term they used for it at that point. I went and hung a wreath on the front of the pub door telling him I was sorry to hear about his upcoming bereavement *(laughs)*. That was his first little hint when he didn't pay. The second one was when I went in and put a pig's head in the middle of his dining room table and emptied a pint of maggots over it in the early hours in the morning.

By the time he got up, it would have been half eaten away *(laughs)*. That was just to let him know that we could get in if we wanted without waking him. He'd already had the wreath and this was his next warning *(laughs)*.

It's a way of saying 'You know who you've got to pay' sort of thing *(laughs)*. This is a tried and tested way. But it's not a nice thing to be doing. I don't like violence. I suppose it's a strange thing to say for somebody who has been in the line of work that I've been in all these years, isn't it? But I don't like it. It's not always necessary *(laughs)*. If you need to use it, then use it, but if it's not needed, then don't. Sort it out by speaking. You don't need to hit anybody *(laughs)*. But no, violence ain't good.

I would never hit a woman. It dates back to they way my dad was with my mum. I would not hit a woman. About the worst I do is smack my step daughter's arse if she's been misbehaving. But that is as far as I will go. I don't agree with violence against women. I have been known to get aggressive with men for being violent with women *(laughs)*. It's one of them situations I do not agree with at all.

The minute most people hear my condition they think of the shower scene in the film 'Psycho'. Paranoid schizophrenic with psychotic tendencies. Then I have to sit there and explain what being psychotic actually means. It's

214

not that I'm going to be running trying to stab everybody. It's just when I'm ill, I retreat into my own make-believe little space. I can't be arsed with normalities of life. I'd rather go and play in my own little world. That's what it boils down to for me really. You see people do a double take when they hear the diagnosis. There's a certain amount of fear. Sometimes that can be a buzz, when you see that look on someone's face *(laughs)*. Other times there's like, you see the look on some of the little kids' faces and stuff and it's not nice. I gripped hold of one little girl, my step-daughter's friend, we'd taken her out and she was just really misbehaving. She was rolling about on the floor at the cinema, so I grabbed her by the shoulders and lifted her bodily to her feet and the look that came across her face was one of pure terror. I don't like that sort of thing *(laughs)*. Sometimes it can be a good thing, sometimes it can be bad. It's not the world's best like, but it has it's good points.

There are lots of people that know about my diagnosis for example, and they know what I'm capable of and will not cause me problems. Their attitude is he can do it and he's mad enough to do it *(laughs)*. It's that simple. A lot of people just don't want to know because they know I've got this diagnosis, which makes life a hell of a lot easier trying to retire *(laughs)*. If I say no I'm not interested, they're more likely to take notice because they don't want to fuck about with a lunatic. That's the way they look at it, you know what I mean? *(laughs)*. So it could be handy in that respect. As I said it has it's good points.

My own little world? Oh I can just put myself there. It's a better world than this one. When I can't be bothered with the real one, when I'm not feeling too good, I go there. Yes, I see things. It's a difficult one to explain. It's like the real world is there, but it's overlaid with my one *(laughs)*. So like if I was in that situation right now, I could be sat in the chair speaking to you, but at the same time I could be holding a conversation with a leprechaun sat on a tree stump in the corner, or something, do you know what I mean? *(laughs)*. I've actually done this with doctors. Sat there telling them what the dwarf or the leprechaun or the elf is saying. It's like an overlap, as if you've got double images on picture, which is scary in it's own way *(laughs)*. But it's a fantasy world. I mean, I realise when I'm getting unwell now. I've had the illness a long time. It's usually a slow build up. Then I do try and get help. There are occasions where it's too late and it's already there. Then it's a case of my missus getting the doctor out. Sometimes it's not nice. It's like tripping on acid, sort of thing. You don't know what's reality and what isn't. Well it could be extremely dangerous in certain circumstances. Say you were cooking food and stuff, it could be really dangerous. Thankfully that hasn't happened yet.

Jackie

Jackie approached me at a talk I was giving about the book. Her sparkly eyes and warm manner drew me to her immediately. A few weeks later we met in her home; a spacious, well-kept house. She spoke easily whilst plying me with drinks and snacks. Jackie will be 61 this year. She has recently applied to become a 'befriender' to the elderly

It happened nearly twenty years ago. My husband said I was sort of high before that, but I mean we didn't really know what high meant back then. He'd say something like 'Are you on cloud nine Jack?' and I'd think 'What's he on about like?' *(laughs)* So there was something there before I had the breakdown. At the time they said it could be a slight form of schizophrenia. They don't really know why it happened. I was down in Wales. I used to go down there when my children were young and stay with my family, for a holiday you see. My hubby would stay at home. One night I'd woken up and where I lay it was though my whole body was on fire. My mind just went off like a rocket. I thought my mother was dying you see. I used to have to listen to her breathing in and out, and this particular time I thought she wasn't. I rushed over to her and woke her up in a state. I was agitated and I was making her scared. It was very emotional. My son was only five and he was trying to help me, because I couldn't keep still, on the couch and all. I couldn't, I just could not keep still. And he sort of said to me, 'Sit on the floor mum'. So I sat on the floor, and he put his blanket around me keeping me warm and sat by me and that. I was very agitated. I believe in the One Above and I was talking to Him. It was all very traumatic.

This happened at four in the morning. My mother lived in sheltered accommodation. Eventually she went over to the warden and asked her to phone for my sister to come down. My sister worked at the hospital; she's not a qualified nurse but she knows a little bit about things. I don't know whether I was frightening my mother but my sister kept saying to her you know, 'just keep calm, keep calm, I'll see to it' like. They took me up to the hospital and I was a bit calmer by then. My cousin worked up there as well. My sister had asked her to come down from her home, to come and stop with me at the hospital as well. Just to be there you know. Eventually I got to see the doctor and I don't know what drivel I was telling him *(laughs)* but it was decided that I'd have to go up to the bigger hospital in Abergavenny. By that time my hubby had come from Worcester and my nieces and nephews were there too. One of them was very strong for me, the other two were upset. They couldn't really do anything, they were so upset. It was a very, very nerve wracking journey to the hospital. I saw the psychiatrist and he said it might be a mild form of schizophrenia. So I was put on medication and had to stop down the psychiatric ward. My hubby took my two children home and he would come and see me at weekends. My sister would come

218

down and see me in that time but I had to stop there and it was terrible. Terrible. I was so agitated.

Now I think that it might have been to do with the sudden death of my father. That it came on through bereavement you know? I was 17 when my father died though, and I had my breakdown aged 39, two months before my fortieth birthday. So there were twelve years in between. But my father was a bandmaster and he had an assistant bandmaster. His assistant bandmaster had a breakdown a fortnight before I did so I think there must be a link in there somewhere. The same month, the same year, but he had his breakdown in the home. He never had to go to hospital or anything. I think it was probably bereavement over my father for him as well. You know it happened to both of us within a fortnight of the same month, the same year. I mean that's more than a coincidence isn't it? Him having a breakdown too. He still hasn't got over it and I don't think he ever will. He was a bag of nerves then and he still is a bag of nerves. My mother suffered with nerves as well and she used to have to go to hospital. She got stomach ulcers. She had to go and spend time in hospital just on a sort of milk diet. My father and my sister never suffered with nerves but I'm a worrier like.

I was in hospital down in Wales for three weeks. I play an instrument and I asked my husband to bring my trumpet down. Occupational Therapy it was you see, you could do what you liked at certain hours. I would play my trumpet. Oh it was lovely surroundings there you know. Beautiful. Beautiful. I used to play my trumpet, and then other patients would hear it outside and say, 'Oh that's lovely that is'. I remember one lady, she was anorexic. I didn't know what anorexia *was* in those days you see. Anyway she clung to me like glue. Other people were saying 'Why don't you eat?' and talking all about food to her all the time. I never mentioned food, and she was my shadow. It was nice but a little bit frightening. I wanted space because I was very ill as well you see. But I stuck it. I didn't tell her to go away or anything. I asked my niece about the anorexia and I said ' How can I help her?' She said 'well ask her to go to the little shop down the road with you'. We were allowed out of the hospital to go to the shop see. So one day I said to her 'If I buy you a packet of crisps will you eat them?' She didn't say anything but I tried it and she ate a couple. Yes. She ate a couple. After that I don't know what happened to her. I came home to England and then I had to go straight back into hospital there.

Perhaps I wasn't really sorted. When I came back after my initial breakdown, they gaveme the medication that I'm still on now. I've been in hospital, about ten times in all *(laughs)*. It is a wonderful place when you need it, but when

220

you're feeling better it's very boring. You should be able to tell them when you want to go home, because each person is different. I say to the nurses, 'put a good word in for me', you know, with the psychiatrist, because they all get around on a Thursday say and have a chat to see who is well enough to go home. Then I come out and I have to strive again, when I come out into society. I've had a few jobs in the past, just cleaning jobs you know, while my son was growing up and that. We managed, but initially after my breakdown my husband and daughter could not handle it. Terrible it was. Terrible. Well I was agitated you see, and snappy. I just wanted them to say something that would soothe me like. Give me a bit of relaxation like. But they didn't know how. So I was trying to help myself and I had to show them how to help me as well, and it didn't always work *(laughs)*. But I stuck at it...*(small laugh)*. There is light at the end of the tunnel. But it's how you get there. It's very, very hard. But I made it and I'm jolly well proud of myself.

Initially they thought it was schizophrenia when I had the breakdown see. But eventually I was diagnosed with manic depression, and I thought 'oh-oh I've got a stamp across my head now. 'Manic Depression'. And I didn't like that...*(laughs)*. You know it's a horrible label. There are no fit words to describe it.

I get so fed up because the only people we hurt are ourselves. We give ourselves a headache, right here. I got so fed up of giving myself a headache from worrying about stupid things. I'd be screwing my eyeballs up. Terrible. Popping out they would be. You know, you worry about something and then you think, oh it was ten years ago that happened and you worry about something else. On and on and on and on. My son has been a pillar of strength. He's absolutely wonderful. He says 'You have not got to worry if you don't want to mam'. Well of course you haven't, but how do you teach yourself not to? We have forgotten how not to worry. Not all illnesses are like that I suppose, I don't really know, but with manic depression it is. It's all worry, worry, worry.

Ouch, the pain sometimes is absolutely terrible. It's like a headache and your eyeballs are throbbing *(laughs)*. You feel like getting them out. That's what I say I want to do. And hitting yourself against a wall. I've done it myself. In the house like. It doesn't hurt because you want the pain to go away so much. You have to stop the pain yourself. You put it there so it's up to you to get it out. By relaxing. By telling yourself not to worry. What can you do if you worry? Nothing. You don't know what's going to happen in a minute. Or next month. If you worry about, say you've got a job interview next week; you'll be thinking, 'Oh no, will I get it?' I mean, even if you worry for a week you still don't know. 'Till you're actually sat down having your interview. You've got to learn that yourself. How not to worry. We have forgotten. You just tell yourself off, punish yourself, instead of saying I'll do it tomorrow. 'Not today', I say sometimes. Well I've got to do something. 'Not today', I say. Then I take a deep breath, 'not today'. It's all relaxation. I mean everyone takes the world, takes their life for granted, but when you have a mental illness, you do not. You have to learn again how to do it. It's easy if you will let yourself have a go. I say you can tell yourself off a hundred times today. Try and tell yourself off ninety-nine tomorrow. At least you'll had one little tiny bit of relaxation. It's worth it. Yes. Really it is.

I know why people bang their head against walls. They want to get rid of the pain, and the *wall* won't let them down. They need support, something that won't let you fall. I told my psychiatrist about this. I said I know why people self-harm. It's because their mind is too busy at that moment when they're worrying and their body is just there. They harm their body, 'cos it's not doing what it's supposed to be doing. Because the mind won't let it. You know, won't let it *walk*, won't let it do *anything* because it's too busy. In the past, I've bitten the backs of my fingers. The skin has had to come off even if it hurts. It really has got to come off because that's my punishment. People self-harm maybe

223

because they've hurt somebody, or they can't forgive themselves. It's a mixture of things. And fear, that's what it is. I told my psychiatrist that. I said to him 'I want to help people', like at the centre I go to, because I love 'em. I just love 'em to bits. I *always* say 'How are you, see?' (I say) 'How are you?' and they say: 'I'm not very well'.

You know it hurts me when they say that. But they're so used to me saying 'How are you?', that they don't think to say 'How are *you* Jackie?' See they're just thinking of … you know what I mean, they're just thinking of themselves. 'How are you?' They're sort of not interacting. I don't know how to explain it. Sometimes, you know, when someone does ask me how I am, I'm so surprised I forget myself. That's just me, see. That's just how I am *(laughs)*. Usually they're so involved with their own thoughts, their own feelings. Yes.

God, worrying. What do I worry about? I worry about everything and then my mind tells me to have a rest. That's when I can't cope outside, you know. I can't cope doing the cooking and all that. So I go into hospital and have a rest. No one, my hubby, nor anybody else hasn't got the right to tell me to go into hospital. I tell me. Nobody else. That's not right. Because in later life you could hate them and think, 'Oh you made me go into hospital.' I decide when I go in and I decide when I come out. 'Cos as I said I came out once and I wasn't ready and I was back in a week later *(laughs)*.

One time I went into hospital - nearly twelve years ago now - when my mother was dying. She was in Wales and I couldn't cope at all. You know, with getting the dinner and all that. Who cares when my Mum is dying? She had cancer. For a fortnight she was hanging on for life, and she was asleep, always asleep. They kept her sedated because of the pain. Cancer of the pancreas she had. She couldn't have any food, she was a skeleton. I went down there for a while but when she went into hospital I had to come back home because I was getting agitated over her being in a hospital and seeing her like that. Then I had to come home and go into hospital myself *(laughs)*. I asked my sister to tell me when my mother died. To phone up the hospital and I'd get the message. And, it was so bad I..., well one of the nurses came, and I said 'If I put my hands out will you take them?', and she said 'yes'. She comforted me she did. By the time I went to the funeral though, I was high as a kite *(laughs)*. That's what it's like with manic depression. But because I didn't seem to be upset no one came to comfort me. My sister was crying all the time and everyone was comforting her. Our house is on a mountain road, and past the last few houses is fields, I went out up the road and I was shouting and crying to the sheep *(laughs)*.

Sometimes when you have depression and that and you're coming out of it, well I personally can't switch my mind off you know. You're talking to someone and your conversation is going alright but when you stop talking, the more you think of; I said that, but I should have said that, or this. Oh that's horrible that is. I'll have to do a mind over matter then. Just walk around doing the washing up or something, with one hand squeezing the washing up brush, just trying to concentrate on that. You know, thinking it *will* go. And then you might think oh well, I can't switch off so what? Shut up and do something else *(laughs)*. It will go eventually. But when you can't switch off it's horrible. You can get really aggressive with yourself you know. But when you do manage it, it feels wonderful, people don't understand how it feels.

Both my children convinced me that you haven't got to worry if you don't want to. Well, you haven't. It's your own thoughts making your body unhappy you know. You feel sorry for yourself, poor old me. Well there's thousands of people out there got it. But it's 'poor old me'. I used to say it you know, 'poor old me' all the time. Now I'm more like well never mind if you've got depression. Hard luck. Get on with it you know. Force yourself to do things because you must keep on the go. Write it down, keep a diary. I don't like it, but it's a good idea *(laughs)*. I've found out a lot of things that can help me though. I do a facial exercise to stop stress. I told my psychiatrist that I can relax by closing one eye at the time. It sounds funny but it works.

When I go up to see him (my psychiatrist), I write what I've got to say down, 'cos otherwise you're there in the waiting room, thinking 'what was I thinking last Thursday?' I'll write it down, and well, then my conscience is clear. I was up there last week and there was a young girl come in. The conversation started because I said that I wrote all my thoughts down. I think it must have been her first time there. She was lovely you know. She was Pakistani and I went over, chatting to her. Muslim she was and she was telling me all about it. It was fascinating. She was so lovely. She was married and she had some rings like. And all these gold earrings, and all these bracelets on. I said

'Which is your wedding ring then?'

'Oh I don't have a wedding ring' she said. 'I have rings of my mother in law and of my mother.'

She had about twelve *(laughs)*. I said, 'Is this putting you off you know, talking to you?' She said, 'No. It's doing me good' she said *(laughs)*.

Doctor James came out and he was running late so he came over and said 'I won't be long Jackie'.

I said 'I'm alright talking to this young lady' *(laughs)*. He's lovely he is. I said - because I've seen him twice now - I said 'Do you think I've got a mental illness?'

227

He said 'Well I've only seen you twice', he said 'but you show no signs of mental ill health'. That made me feel good and I told him that I'd made a complete recovery. And the psychologist said I was unique. I thought 'Damn me I am' *(laughs)*.

I said to the doctor 'How can I help people?'

He said 'you're already doing it Jackie'. Now I never heard anything else when he said that, because he bought tears to my eyes. He was so sentimental. He's so confident of his job. I said, 'You're a smashing doctor'.

He says 'I'm only doing my job'.

I said 'Yes, but you're doing a thorough good job of it'.

I mean he's just got a little office by the fire exit. You know, his door is a fire exit *(laughs)*. He sits there with his comfy chair and he's really relaxed, you know. Because if you go to a psychiatrist and you've got a table there between you both, phew, that ain't no good. Frighten you to death. Like the old Headmaster. It's got to be casual. Laid back. One to one, but not under those circumstances where they've got a white coat on. Oh god no. I went somewhere one time and they had white coats on. Oh God, I mean that was terrible. I was singing 'They're coming to take me away' *(laughs)*. High I was.

I've never worried about paying bills or anything like that 'cos my hubby is as good as gold. This house was ours from the day we bought it. We won twelve thousand pounds on the coupons. We were very, very lucky. Every fork, every knife, every spoon was paid for. Wonderful. Wonderful it was. We've been here thirty-five years now nearly. It's nice isn't it? I wanted to make it all nice for you to come, to welcome you.

My hubby has got a bit of a temper on him. He's mellowed over the past few years. He's more understanding now. Which is nice. Of course, in the past I was afraid of him see. You know he's got a terrible temper and it will flare up (clicks her fingers) just like that, over anything. You know he would say something to me and I would take all those words to heart. He knew I was afraid of him, but now I can stick up for myself. Because I've learnt, and I ain't going to take it anymore. He never hurt me physically, only mentally. I haven't got to put up with it anymore and since I've shown him, he's given me more respect and more love. I didn't have to put up with it. 'Cos it was hurting me and he'd got no right. Nobody's got the right to touch my finger if I don't want them to. I know about people who get abused and all. And with, rape you know, I think I know the feeling of being raped. It's terrible you know, interference with your body. Something different that's not supposed to be, pushed onto you. You haven't got to take it. Then you've got to learn to relax again. You know, absorb the pain and then get rid of it. It takes time and patience.

He didn't abuse me physically but he abused me mentally, mentally. Yes it was terrible, terrible. I used to feel not worthy and think 'Oh I can't do nothing'. Because he'd tell me off all the time. If I don't do it, he'll tell me off. See and if I'd do it, he will too. I mean once I'd gone down to Wales when the kids were little. With a baby. I had to pack the cot, I've had to pack clothes and the towels, and everything else going, and nappies and pins and all that. And my hubby used to go out for a drink every night with my brother-in-law when we were there, see. When it came to him cleaning his teeth, I had to pack again and we had to come home. Because I'd forgotten the toothbrush. He wasn't willing to buy a toothbrush down in Wales.

He's English. He's a cabinet maker – he made that one over there see. When I, when we first got married and someone would come to our house and ask him to make something for him, I had to leave the room. I wasn't allowed to be involved with his friends from England because I was from Wales. I'm positive that had something to do with it. He was jealous. All jealousy. I mean, I never brushed him away from any part of my home down in Wales. From my friends. You know he was always involved. But even when my mother used to come down for holidays, she would have to go out. And my auntie, she had to go out of my home too, if someone else came in about a job for him. He was terrible.

He was jealous for some reason. I don't know why. He was a friend of the family, so I'd known him years and years. He used to come down and stay with us. As I say we won £12,000 and we come to live here. We could have had a good life. But he was terrible, terrible. I think it had something to do with making me ill. I don't hold grudges though. Someone said to me recently, 'What's your husband like?' I said 'well he's bald on top, he wears glasses, wears a hearing aid, and I love every inch of him.'

I truly mean that now. Not many people would say that after thirty-four years and how he used to be. But I love him. I look at him and I think, 'he's all mine', you know *(laughs)*. I mean I don't know his thoughts because I'm not a bloke you know. And he don't know mine because he's not a woman. And this is how love is. You have to work at it... *(pause)*. Mental illness doesn't have to affect love. Not in my experience anyhow.

A lot of people have helped me, you know. Sometimes when you don't expect it. One time when I was going to band every Tuesday night - my hubby would take me because I can't drive - and I was very agitated. I've found out that if I go to band it takes my mind off things see. It takes my mind away from home and things see. This one time though I didn't want to go I was so agitated, and all of a sudden we slowed down in the traffic, and out of the corner of my eye I saw a tandem, coming past with a father and a daughter or what have you on it. And I suddenly thought 'right, yes, life, this is life.' It clicked into place. You've got to go on. It's got to go on whatever. That moment was good, it was right. It felt right. And I went to band and came home happy. I do love playing in the band see. As I said my late father was a band master and both my sister and I were in a band when we were growing up.

I always had hope that I would get better. Yes. Yes always. If I could do it once I could do it another time. I went into hospital once and I don't know how many days I was in for but I went to the loo and there was a mirror. I looked at myself and my face looked like a stewed prune, all screwed up. And I thought I don't want to be like this for much longer *(laughs)*. I learnt to do things to make me relax. Keep me calm. I've had...I mean I had a relaxation tape. That generally saved my life it did. One day I was so agitated. There was no breeze outside. Everything was still. And I couldn't find a corner of my home where I could get relief. I felt like a caged animal. I was suicidal there. God I could of gone to the river and chucked myself in but I'm afraid of the water. I thought 'I ain't going to do it that way, I don't like the water' *(laughs)*. So I went upstairs looking for my tape, and when I found it I was still agitated. I wanted this tape to start. I'd got this tape like, and it wouldn't start, and then it was on the wrong side, and patience is a virtue and all that, you know, take it out, look at it, try it again, and again and 'are there any batteries?' and 'is the electric plugged in?', and then I was laying on my bed and that man saved my life.

I wanted to kill myself, for it to stop. I mean I don't know whether I would of gone through with it but I felt it, the vibes were certainly there. That's the one time I remember. I just lay there while this bloke came on telling you to relax your body, you know, every muscle like, and it calmed me. He literally saved my life. I must have put it in the washing machine recently with the clothes see, 'cos I've buggered it up *(laughs)*. I need a new one. But I play my instrument and I sing and that calms me as well. My neighbour is out most of the time so he's not disturbed and he wouldn't tell me off anyway *(laughs)*. But ah, God, I try to sort it out; to calm myself. Aargh dear. It's finding a middle. I love my home see, and sometimes when you're out, you want to be at home. But then sometimes when you're home, you want to be out. You can't get a middle.

I'm on lithium. It has helped me in the past but last year, I told my psychiatrist - one of the chaps I see - that before I'm 60 next year, I want to be off my tablets. And he laughed at me. I don't know whether it was a snigger or not, but I feel I was laughed at. Anyhow I saw him again and he said 'Are you really serious about reducing your medication?', and I said 'I am'. So I've reduced it, in one year I've reduced it by half. My body is telling me with side effects that I don't need it anymore you see. I have nausea; when I come down in the morning, I feel terrible. And I feel giddy sometimes. I slur my words, I can't get a sentence out sometimes. I've really got to concentrate. The calves of my legs are itching all the time. It's the side effects you get from your tablets see. It tells you about them with the list you get with them, that those side effects are amongst them. I never used to get them though. I went to the psychiatrist last week, or a fortnight ago or something, I said 'I want to reduce them again'. He said 'Well you know I don't really like to reduce them in case you go too high or low'. I said 'don't worry about that' I said, 'I ain't going anywhere. I've been there I don't like it.' So we reduced them to half and we'll see how it goes and then in six months reduce it some more. I'll be off them by next year. I don't like taking them. It's only a swallow, but I hate it. I don't think I need it anymore.

I worked in halls of residence for about four years. I was a cleaner. When I first went there, the boss at that time had a mental illness as well and everything was lovely for those few years. Then a new boss came, a younger boss and he found out I had a mental illness. I don't know how he found out, he must have chatted to the staff or what have you. But he wanted me out. My hubby's a union man and he told me they wanted to get me out first because I'd been there the longest. I asked the boss, you know, did the other boss tell you I suffered with mental illness before you started like. He said 'Yes'. He used to get me down to come down the office, 'Come down to the office Jackie', 'What have you been doing?'.

'I had to wash blankets off the bed. Look.'
The washing machine was downstairs, out at the back and I'd had to go out there. I said I'd been washing the blankets. But the washing machine didn't always work properly and I had to go back down, halfway through to make sure everything was working alright. Then I had to go back down again and put it in the tumble dryer. I told him all this. He said 'But you were seen here'. I said yes, I had to take my hoover up and take my bucket up, and all that while I was doing the top floor. And they had carpets on the stairs. Then he said 'you were in the toilet for quarter of an hour.' I was told that I was walking around the building in a daze.

Now if I'd been walking around the building in a daze, I wouldn't have been going to work. I'm not stupid enough to do that. They put me off on the sick and told me that they felt I couldn't do my job. So I had to wait until my husband came in and signed a form with me to say that they could go and ask my doctor about my state of health. My mental state of health. The doctor came back and said 'she's perfectly able to her job', you know dusting and hoovering and all that. It ended up with them deciding that they had to have me back again. I ended up in a terrible state. My CPN nurse came to see me, and I went to see the psychiatrist and I ended up in a terrible state. The day I had to go back, I just did not want to, I did not want to get up. I shuffled my feet along the road going there. I knew they'd be putting me down, or I don't know what. I was watched, you know, really watched I was. I was watched all the time.

And then, they came again and said 'And what have you been doing Jackie?' You know again, 'We think you're not doing your job properly.'

'Well what happens now?' I said.

'Well we think you're not doing your job properly. And we've had complaints off the residents.'

I said, 'Oh no you haven't. Nobody would complain about me because I'm like a bloody mother hen. I'm like a mother hen over there.' I'm like 'Hello. How are you? I've done your room.' Or 'What do you want me to do to your room?' 'Good as gold I am.' I said   They must of thought 'oh no Jackie's not falling for this one'.

So I said 'what happens now?'

He said, 'One verbal. Then another verbal and then the sack.'

Well I wasn't gonna have that, waiting, just waiting. My hubby said 'Jack, whatever you do, do not walk out.' But I thought well I can't take this, you know. I ain't gonna wait for them to come around and tell me to go. I had the keys to the rooms and I said 'shove 'em'.*(laughs).* So I came home and I felt jolly well better. They said 'We'll have to send you a letter to say that you've thrown your keys at me and you do realise that you've lost your job like.' I said yes. Phew. The relief was absolutely marvellous.

My hubby said 'write down everything that's happened'. I wrote it all down; the dates and the times of all these things that happened and we went to the advice bureau. A woman there got in touch with the union bloke and I took them as far as you know, not into court but I took them as far as court, or whatever they call it – a tribunal, that's it. The chap, the union bloke said, 'Look I can't be on your side or their side you know, when we sort it out.' I was on holiday in Scotland and they phoned me up and said 'Are you willing to settle. They're don't want you to go to court'.

I said 'How much will they give me?'

She said 'Minimum 500 quid'. So that's all I had. I was told afterwards I could have had thousands.

My psychiatrist had given me a letter to say there was nothing wrong with me. Saying this stress was from what they were giving me. It was just terrible. So I thought well 500 quid. While I was waiting for the cheque, I thought this is my blood money. I don't want it now. I don't want this. I could have chucked it away easily. I never touched it for twelve months. It was in the old bank you know. Giving me a bit of interest *(laughs)*. But after about a year I started to spend it. I began to think 'why not?'.

I go to a daycentre now. The ladies who worked there before the two who are there now were excellent. But the ladies there now, they do not integrate. The only pleasure they have is ... well is coming in with a list and bag to get our dinner money. It's absolutely terrible. And we're hassled every Wednesday to have a meeting. We're hassled! Hassled. 'Come on now, we're having the meeting now'. You know . When there's 'Anybody got any other business', nobody will say nothing. I'm fed up of it. So I don't know whether to say anything. I think I'm just going to let them get on with it 'cos I'm going to leave soon. I don't need it see. Don't need it. All my friends are there though and I think the world of them. I help them. There's a lady there who doesn't know sometimes whether she wants to go to the loo now or in a minute. She can't decide. And I'm there, you know saying, 'have a cup of tea, sit down' when she comes into the room. She's frightened too sometimes. Although she sees the same old people there every week, something in her mind is telling her that this is not right, or whatever, I don't know. But I'll coax her, say sit down you know. I wait on her, get her a cup of tea, sit with her till she's comfortable. Now those girls should be doing that. Somebody said to me, 'You were doing their job Jackie'. And I ain't getting paid for it. I'm doing it for love. But ah....and the other one who works there, she ain't that good either.

There are wonderful people around though. I have met a heck of a lot of wonderful people, in my nineteen years. And that's from psychiatrists down to users. They have been some absolutely marvellous people. Who would not hurt a fly. They wouldn't truly. Some service users are wonderful. For example, there was a lady sat down and a gentleman by the side of her and she was, looking for her money to pay for food like, and some money went down in between the seats and he said 'Oh look, you've dropped some money here', and he got the cushions for her and looked for it, found it and gave it to her back. You know, they wouldn't steal off anyone. They wouldn't.

We lost a lady recently. A lady from the centre. She died last week and the funeral is this week, so we're all upset at the moment like. I mean she was getting on in years but it don't matter. She'd had a phobia for fifty-odd years about bathrooms. And her hands were white, from her washing them all the time. All the time she'd wash them. All the time. Once she came in agitated and I said

' How are you?'

'Oh not very well'.

Then she put her hand tight on mine and she said 'What can I do my dear?

'I don't know' I said. 'I truly don't know how to help you'.

She just let go. 50 odd years she'd had this. She was talking with the psychologist about it, and she said that - I don't know whether this caused it or not - but when she was little, about eight years old, one of her friends dies, and a mother said not to play with her - this lady - to some other children because she caused the death of this friend. I don't know whether I got that right, but it was like someone told her she was dirty. She carried that with her through her whole life. You know, she couldn't go in anyone's bathroom. She didn't live far away from mine, fortunately, so she could go home to go to the loo like. Then one time she had diarrhoea you know and she messed herself. So she stopped eating, she wouldn't eat anything. She was so embarrassed about it and thought she was dirty. It didn't matter you know but to her it did. It was very, very frightening for her. Terrible (long pause).

I'm involved in the mental health network here and they're talking about people having a paid job to teach the media about mental illness. I don't know how they go about it, and they say they have the money to do it but we have to wait for a meeting in a few months, to see what will happen. I said I would help out in that way you know. So I'm waiting to hear about that. As I've said I'm a hundred and ten percent for mental health. I've experienced it, I've learnt and I've come through, and I want to show other people how good it can be. Because it is an absolutely wonderful life. Everyday is different. I mean people's lives change, of course, but mine has changed enormously. How I can sit here feeling relaxed and thinking well this is good, just talking to you, and when you've gone, I've got to do whatever, but at the moment, just for this moment, I'm talking to you. Don't matter about this morning, and don't matter about yesterday, because that's gone. Can't do nothing about it, if anybody said anything to hurt you or you took it the wrong way, hard luck *(laughs)*. It don't matter, because if you hold onto that you're hurting yourself for no good reason, it's not necessary. Not necessary. I've done it myself plenty of times.

I said to my son when I saw him today, he was here when I got in. I'd been down the town like, I came home, and he's got a car and it was parked there in the front. I thought 'I recognise that car numberplate', you know, 'I recognise that one'. He's still got a front door key see. He's an assistant, he's training to be a manager. A trainee manager he is. He had to go to court today to get a license, under his name or something in the shop or whatever see. He wears a suit there so he's all posh. I come in and he came down from the loo.

He said 'Are you alright mam?'

I said 'Yes'.

'Is everything alright?' he says:.

I said 'yes. I'm so happy' (*laughs*).

Sometimes if I keep on saying I'm so happy, they tell me to shut up see. They don't realise how wonderful it feels, so I learnt that I don't say, 'oh I feel happy' like too often. But I said it to him, and if he'd shut me up or was sort of 'Oh mam don't go on', I'd accept it. And today he gave me a kiss and a hug. I said 'what are you doing here like?'. He told me he had to go to court. I said 'When have you got to be back?' He said 'now'. So don't keep me talking sort of (*laughs*). He said 'I only came to go to the loo and have a drink'.

My daughter still lives with me. Her boyfriend didn't have any good job prospects but they're getting better. So she'll want to move out soon. Sometimes she does house-sitting. When her friends go away and you know, they trust her, which is nice. To stop at their home. She was doing that about a fortnight ago and I really missed her. I've never missed her before. But I missed her and I told her. She said 'Oh its nice to be missed' (*laughs*).

She wants to leave but 'cos of the price of houses and all this, it's hard. But she wants to leave and that's that. She says, 'Oh I wish I could win the lottery.' And I say to myself, 'well the Lord can't do miracles. You have to do those yourself' (*laughs*). Her turn will come though. My son's not married but he's left home, and he doesn't come round that much see. And when he does come around, after a while, I think well I wish he'd go home now *(laughs)*. I don't know why I do that. I don't say it like, but I wish he'd bugger off (*laughs*). When my daughter leaves she'll be coming back a lot more times than him. That's the way it is with girls. She's on permanent nights at work at the moment to get a bit more money. She's taken holiday this week and she's with her boyfriend. It will all work out alright in the end. And I want my house to myself again. 'Cos we only had it twelve months before she came on the scene. It's thirty-two years later I want my house back (*laughs*). I'll have it back one day.

Steve

Steve came across as gentle but extremely troubled at times. Thirty-five years old, he had been taking heroin since the age of twelve. He received a diagnosis of schizophrenia in 1993, following a drug-induced psychosis. When I interviewed him he had been clean for 16 months.

I haven't seen my dad since I was four. I've got a photograph of him that my mum had in a drawer, that I keep in a frame. When he left I went to foster parents. I was there for about a year. Then I was put into a secure unit sort of thing in Bristol. For maladjusted children. Social Services had said my Mum couldn't cope with me. Anyway I was there for about a year, then they realized that I wasn't as much a danger as they had first thought and put me into a boarding school. I was in boarding school for about ten and a half years till I was 16 and a half.

I'd been out of school for about six months when I first got in trouble with the police and I was brought up in front of the courts. It was a shock to get arrested and it messed up my life completely. Coming home in the holidays I used to use drugs, go back to school and clean myself up. Mainly heroin. But from the first day I left school, I started using and it became a habit. Before that it had only been recreational.

Then in '91, no in 1986, I went to a Young Offenders Institution. I done 12 months there, left there, done two and a half years on the streets. Fighting, getting into trouble and that sort of thing. I went to main prison '91. I was in and out of prison '91-'93. It was in prison that my friends gave me an acid tab. I was out of my cell, everything was sweet you know, all laughing and joking, it was really good. Then everyone was banged up and I was put back in my cell. I couldn't get my head round this acid tab, it just made me really depressed. Really withdrawn. That was the start of my mental illness, I think. I started hearing voices coming out of the vents and I thought they were in the cell. So I'm up there with my lighter, looking through vents and I couldn't see nothing. Then I started to hear my name on the radio, people like saying I'm this, I'm that, horrible things. I started hearing them more and more. I was also getting flashbacks of the prisoners and the officers laughing and joking about me. I didn't know what to do. I was troubled. I'd never experienced the voices before and I thought they was real. I had these pictures in my head; flashbacks of the screws laughing at me.

While this was going on I'd gone to court to receive the charges I was up for and they gave me bail. I managed to get into a hostel in Bristol. I was still hearing voices, still really troubled and I didn't know what to do. I'd never experienced this before. The voices were saying things like 'We've phoned the police', 'We're going to bury you', 'We're going to shoot you'. I was getting photograph pictures in my mind of the Filth. Then I got a voice saying 'there's people coming. They're gonna take you away and going to dispose of you and that's it'. So I'm hearing this and I'm hearing other voices telling me I'm no good and stuff. Then there's a knock on the door and there's two friends that I know from Bath. I'm automatically thinking, 'They're here. Fuck, they've come to take me away and they're gonna dispose of me'. So like…I'm not well and my head just goes. I just lost it. My friends seen how troubled I was and how different I was from the last time they saw me. They couldn't understand what was wrong. They had a go at the staff at the hostel saying, 'What have you done to him? He was such a happy-go-lucky person. He really liked being at the centre of everything like, always laughing and joking.' I'd gone back to the room, saying to them 'I can't speak to you, I can't see you, go.' I'd gone back into my room and had like a nervous breakdown sort of thing. My friends got back to Bath that evening and they'd gone round and seen my sister, and told her about the state I was in.

My sister phones up and speaks to the staff and within about half an hour there's a doctor there and they section me for, well, I ended up doing 7 months in a psychiatric ward. Then I was put into a secure unit in Bristol where they gave me Stelazine and I got well. They're telling me that it might be a one–off, that it may not happen again. But it did happen again. I was in jail for burglary at this point and I got a medical discharge to go into hospital. At first I was stealing to get heroin, then I was stealing to get heroin to self-medicate. Anyway in prison they gave me a medical - I don't know what they call it - I think it's a medical discharge thing. Even though I was serving a prison sentence, they put me into a secure unit and I was sectioned. Obviously I can't be released from jail or the secure unit until my time's up. Anyway I broke out of there, tried to hang myself and was found by a security guard. He took me back to hospital. Then they took me back to prison because I chased one of them nurses down the corridor, the voices were there, saying he was running me down and that. I wanted to take his eyes out.

About 3 months later I got put into a medium secure unit: a hospital up in Yorkshire. I done 4 months in there and they said I'm well. But then it took another 3 months to get out of there because Home Office had changed over from Conservative to Labour at the time so I had to wait till when the Home Office, when the Home Office person was to look at my case and say 'well he's safe so we'll release him'. I got well quite quickly there because they gave me drugs; a depot injection in the bum. First every fortnight, then about every month.

I went to a hostel in Bristol and I'd been out of hospital for 10 days when I got caught for burglary and I was put inside for another 2 years. I was burgling to get money, to get the heroin, to get rid of the voices. Self-medicating they call it. I didn't call it self-medicating. I just...do you know what I mean?...it just helped. It just helped. All I know is that it did help with the voices. *(pauses)*... I don't know, it sort of like, I mean it just...Well, when I'm on it I haven't got a care in the world. When I'm on heroin and they're talking to me, I just don't care. I don't care because I've got this heroin inside me and everything's rosy like. When I do come off it, it just goes back to, even worse like, you know what I mean. Heroin takes your mind off stuff for a while. The voices and that. The hallucinations and that. At the time like. When I haven't got any heroin it just wears me down. I just couldn't cope no more. I came to the end of my tether. Sometimes I'd think if I kill myself then I'm not going to get any more of these voices, telling me not to do things. I can't eat because the food's dirty, I'm not allowed to use the toilet because it's dirty. I can't eat food because it's dirty. I mean I can't write letters because I look, well I see into them too much right. So I'm writing letters and they would be quite bizarre. To me you know, what they're saying is real. But to a normal person – if there is such a thing as a normal person – they may think it's a bit bizarre.

Before they put me into a medium secure unit up in Yorkshire, they put me in a forensic hospital and they gave me this injection, that put me to sleep and they put like these things on my head and put electric treatment in my head. Electric shock therapy, ECT, it's called. They gave me 6 loads of it and I didn't feel any different. Looking back now though, I think it messed up my long-term and short-term memory. Scrambled my head like. But it's not as bad as the olden days where they used to give you lobotomies. I feel though that I didn't deserve that electric shock treatment. I didn't have any choice because I was under the Home Office at the time. I had no choice about it.

I was lucky because at the hospital I was in, in Bristol, well one of the staff there took a real interest in me as a person and came to visit me. Said 'I'll help you to get out but you've got to help yourself.' So...um I said OK I will. I was going to get my medication, I was getting my injections. He seen I was helping myself, so this person, this member of staff, said 'we'll get you out.' Then I got bail to go to Bridge House which is in St Paul's in Bristol. Anyway he sees me in, sees me set up and when I'd been clean for a year he says 'I do half days at this house in Darton, in Bristol. Would you like to come there?' I wasn't sure really.

He said 'Well just come and give it a go. Come for a look around and if you like it we'll arrange for you to come and have an assessment.' I agreed and I went there and I liked it, I really did. It was out of the way in a clean area, all the heroin dealers and the crack dealers had been chased out of town, because the community actually got up and said they'd had enough with these people who sell heroin.

I was clean for about two years and I led a normal life. I visited my mum once every month. And my sisters. My sister has stuck by me through thick and thin like, from '93 up 'til now. I was keeping in contact. I was having a few beers but it's not a problem, the beer. I've never had a problem with drinking, you know what I mean? I've seen my mum get beat up by my step-dad, the husband that she's with now, and I think 'I'm not going down that road'. But yeah, I was having a few drinks. About three pints a day. The voices did stop because I was on Modecate and Olanzapine and I was on that for about 5 years. They said then I should have been receiving a review every 12 months but I didn't. They would just give me the injection, give me my pills. It was a case of 'See you later. Come back in 28 days.' But I kept it going, I kept myself clean, had a few beers. No problem. Everything was really smart and then I got this letter from the council saying 'we got a flat for you, down in Bath. Would you like to come and see it?' So I went and saw it but my heart wasn't into it. I look back at it now and my heart wasn't into it. I had this flat for two years, I spent three grand on it, I wasn't using. I managed to save some money – I got a bit of DLA and I saved that, my flat was really nice, but my heart wasn't in it.

Then I started to hear voices again and I became troubled. I started using heroin, I'd been trying for about a year to get on the methadone prescription but it wasn't forthcoming so I had to use. One evening I'm in a friend's house and this guy comes in and says "Scuse me mate. Can you come outside?' So I went outside and these guys attacked me. Broke my nose, cracked my ribs, scuffed up my face, blacked my eyes. Chucked me in the back of a van, took me to this lady's house and said 'Is this the person that burgled your house?' She said 'yes'. They give me another slap, put me in the back of a van. They were going to dispose of me in the woods and that but these other guys came along and said 'Nah. Take him to the police'. And these two people took me into the police station and said, 'He's burgled my mum's house'. I said 'I haven't, I don't know nothing about it.' But they arrested me, they took my trainers off me, and I went into prison. I'm in prison for 6 weeks and I goes to court one day and they says 'we're dropping the charge'.' My solicitor says 'Well, why are you dropping the charge?'. He said 'because the footprints we got doesn't match Mr Jones'. I'd been inside for five weeks for something I haven't done. Anyway in those five weeks they've gone and been through everything else and they'd got me on a camera robbing a shop of alcohol, so that justified the five weeks I'd already spent in jail.

So they've dropped the charge and they were gonna drop the other charges. Then the crown prosecution said that they wouldn't oppose bail so long as I wasn't in Bath or Bristol. My probation officer said there's a hostel in Oxford that might have a place soon but didn't at the moment. They came to an agreement that when a bed came up at this place in Oxford I'd be released and sent there. I've been here ever since *(laughs)*.

I haven't got very many memories of when I was very young and in the secure unit. There were bars like on the window and I know there was a blue light that they kept on at night-time. They used to come round every half hour, every ¾ hour at night to check that we were still there. It was like a secure unit though – doors locked, staff went round with, not chains, but like thin plastic strips with wire through it and their keys, and they used to always walk around with them.

I can remember this one guy; his name was Vincent. Me and him found a window once that wasn't locked, so like we managed to get out the window and gone along a ledge. We're out and we're about five, six like and we come to this pond and we're looking at that and then we goes out onto the road and were grabbed by the night watchman who takes us back. Vincent had a pocket full of goldfish from the pond and he's put tissues in the bottom of the showers and let all these goldfish out*(laughs)*.

I can remember them chucking me into the deep end of a swimming pool as well. I'm on the bottom of the pool and I've come to the top. They're going 'swim' and ever since then I've been able to swim. I couldn't before. They just grabbed me and chucked me in. They used to have like, they used to have like this cupboard and I used to get up there because there was loads of lego in it and at the time I really liked lego. I used to just go up into like this loft cupboard; a little cupboard and I'd go up and there would be loads of lego. I used to spend hours up there.

I can't remember lots of things about though. I *(pauses)*.....and the things I don't remember, I don't know if it was just too bad and I've just blanked it. I can't remember about the food. I cannot remember if we had to go to a dining room. I mean something's happened to blank that out, it may've been good, it may've been bad but I just cannot remember where I used to eat my food. It really puzzles me because, I just, in my head I just cannot remember.

They used to be very strict anyway. If you got caught swearing or anything like that, they put you in this like cage thing. You'd have to laps in it. Well it was about twice the size of this room, and it was tarmacked and all around it, it had a fence. It was all the way around it, except for like a little gate that you'd go in through. If you're naughty, you'd have to go in there and you'd have to do laps as punishment. If they tell you to run, you have to run, if they tell you to walk, you have to walk and if you don't do it you just get given more and more laps and you have to spend more time in there. So I towed the line in there.

There was some good parts about it, there was some nice stuff happening. There was some nice staff who'd say I don't care about the rules, I'm taking this person out and we're going to go and have a walk through the meadows, and see the horses and eat something and do a bit of scrumping like, as you do you know.

One of the memories I had when I first went there was that this guy just come up to me, and it still puzzles me - this guy comes up to me and he gives me this parcel - inside there's this action man, there's sweets and there's all this, all this stuff. I dunno. I still dunno why this this person give me that? I was with a member of staff and everything. To this day I don't know why this person come up to me. It really puzzles me. I don't know why this person has done that.

I used to hide all the time, because I hated it. I... I got a problem with too many people in a room. I can get a bit, a bit*(pauses)*...I don't know what they call it. Anyway, I used to hide and that so I didn't have to do class work. It was all new to me being put away there. I think maybe hiding was some sort of rebellion, on my behalf, because I didn't like it there. I wouldn't tow the line. I didn't wanna be there. I wanted to be home with my mum, I wanted to be home with my sisters, I wanted to be with my brother. I think I decided, well I'm not doing anything they say. I missed my family.

After they said I wasn't as dangerous as what they first thought, my mum still couldn't cope with me, so I had to go away to boarding school. I think part of the reason was that she had three daughters, my three sisters before me and then she had my younger brother, who's a year younger than me. She had like five children and I don't think she could cope. Mum says once I tried to cut this girl's head, some woman's head or something, with an axe once. I did used to scream and cry a lot. And I tried to stab somebody with a knife. I was about five. This boy was about eight or nine and he was hassling us. I missed his heart but the knife's gone into him.

Mum couldn't cope with me because I was 'um lighting fires, smashing everything up. I wouldn't do that, I wouldn't do this. I put it down to my mum and dad splitting up. I was with my dad for the first four years of my life. And then mum split up with up with dad. I think it was that, I wanted my dad – this is what I put it down to – I put it down to I never had my dad. Mum says it's nothing to do with that. She says 'Oh don't be so stupid' but that is what I put it down to. For the first four years I had my dad, then they split up and I wanted him back.

My Mum married my step-dad and 'um he just used to treat me like shit. He used to suffocate me, give me blowbacks of hash and I think he spiked me with LSD as well. I'm sure he did. I must have been about four or five. I can definitely remember him giving me blow backs of hash. He tried to do it one day and at that time I'd broken my arm. I'd said to my sister I'll go and do a somersault and you hold my arm and steady me when I go over and then let go. So I'm jumping and I goes over and she doesn't let go, so I snap my arm and break it. Anyway I got my arm in plaster, a full plaster from elbow to my hand. So when my step dad next tried to give me hash, I hit him over the head with this cast. He was quite shocked but it never happened again after that.

He used to make mashed potato with mustard. To this day, none of my family like it. There was this can of mustard, yellow mustard powder and he used to make a big pan of mashed potato and put loads of this powder in it. Then he'd sit us down and we'd have to stay there, stay there, stay there, until it was gone. If we didn't eat it we couldn't leave. I wouldn't eat it though, I didn't give a shit. He could do what he liked to me, I wasn't eating it. My little brother though, my little brother's a bit naive and he ate it all really quickly. So then he made my brother eat a whole loaf of bread, a plate of chips, baked beans on toast loads of stuff. He made my brother eat all this - he was sick in the end -all because my brother said 'Oh dad look at me'. He didn't realize at that time our real dad had gone, he thought my step-dad was his dad:

'Oh Dad, I've finished it. Aren't I clever?'

'What do you mean you little shit?'

He made him eat all that. My brother had such a hard time off him. He doesn't like talking about it now though. I try to speak to him about it sometimes but he just doesn't want to know. I mean he probably had a horrible life. Obviously most of the time I wasn't there.

The school I went to well, I spent ten and a half years there. At sixteen and a half I wanted to become a vet but the school said I'd spent the maximum amount of time there and I had to leave. For the first three years that I'd

257

been there I didn't go home. For three years I didn't see my family. I wasn't allowed to go home. I missed them yeah very much. But I...I learnt to like my own company. You know I really used to like my own company. They had like 600 acres of land sort of thing. There was a big manor house which was the school building. I used to spend most of the time up in the woods, making dens and bird watching and nesting, climbing trees. I couldn't spell my own name at twelve though, there was no education. It was all, what I call playtime. One thing that bothers me when I look back was that there was about 60 other people in this school and I think well why wasn't it picked up on and me told 'Come on. Come on and join in with the school. Come and have fun with the other children and play.' I didn't have any friends there.

I was abused in school. By the staff. And the other pupils. But I got blanks, blanks, blanks. So I don't know if it's me trying to remember things or if it's nothing.
I know that a teacher used to do it. Used to cuddle me and he used to be sexual and I used to feel very dirty. Really troubled by it. Other people would be like it sometimes as well. I don't know if I was buggered but if I think about it, well my mind's blank now, so I don't know. I don't know what he's done, this one teacher. I did tell the headmaster about this teacher and he didn't do nothing about it. He didn't want to believe it was going on, he said I was making it up. When

I come up here though I said to myself, after my court appearance, I said 'I'm never going back to jail.' I made that promise to myself, my kids, my Mum and my family. And I thought if I'm going to do it properly, get a clean slate, I need to get everything sorted out in my life. I went to the police about the abuse and told them about it and they said that I'd left it too long. I'm trying now just to let it be and to cope with it. I've done all I can really. I know it's gonna be a problem for me for the rest of my life. But the way I look at it, everybody has to cope with things like that in life. I mean there's always things in life that we can't deal with. But it's not worth *(pauses)* ...dwelling over them, do you know what I mean? I was told by the police that they probably, that the person who abused me has probably got a family now. The teacher I mean, or they could be dead now, it's been what twenty years, twenty-five years? Um...it's made me feel a bit depressed. I don't want to think about it too much to tell you the truth. I try to blank it out and try to move on. When I think about it, I try to make myself think of other things so I don't have to.

It used to be an OK school though. We used to go on holidays, to Devon, we'd go to France and we'd go to Scotland. I used to like that. Camp out at nights. Big fires. Most of the time it was alright you know.....But for the first, I think it was three or four years or something I couldn't go home. Everybody else used to go home but not me. Social

Services had said that I needed to grow up, hoping I'd grow out of all my fits and fighting and stuff. Like that if I'd stayed at school and got looked after, I'd be OK.

I still feel angry with my mum. She says she didn't ask to sign over my care. But...Social Services, all Social Services, haven't got no rights to take me and put me in school unless my mum signs over my care I don't think. And I hate thinking about that and I hate her for that. You know I spent ten years at boarding school. I've got no bonds with my family. Didn't know anything about my brothers and sisters except for the holidays I used to have with them*(pauses)*... And I just feel really, really pissed off with my mum...but obviously it's not her fault. She had my other three sisters, then she had my brother, and then a daughter, another girl, and then she had another one, a girl. So there's seven of us in our family, nine altogether with my mum and step-dad. It must have been too much, I mean I was too much of a handful. Especially for her. It was the best thing for her. Once I caught my sister in the eye and I nearly took her eyes out. I used to smash things. I used to be a right git really. Like I say I put that down to not having my dad.

I got my own children now like. I met my ex-partner, it was in '86, I think. I was playing pool and I hit the pool ball and it fell on the floor and this girl came along and picked it up. I looked at her and she looked at me and I asked her if she wanted a game of pool. I was smitten after that night. It was definitely love at first sight. I was with her for sixteen years. We had two children. Obviously I'd done quite a lot of prison in the last nine years I was with her, no in the last twelve really. I was never there, do you know what I mean? I was never home. I was home for, it was almost like holidays *(laughs)*. I'd come home for a holiday, then I'd go back to jail. Obviously I know where she's coming from. Like she said, the children need a stable home. And they need their dad. They need a father, not a part-time dad.

I got a letter off her once when I was in jail. It said 'I'm getting married. We're going to live in Cyprus. I've met somebody else. We're getting married. We're going to live in Cyprus, because he's in the army.' That really screwed my head up. I just couldn't cope with it. It's OK now though. I get to see the children. She doesn't...you know what I mean, she doesn't...she just wanted to make a go of things. She's heard that I'm doing well like. Been clean for a year, well longer than that, sixteen months. And she sees me making an effort like. So that's good.

When I was first diagnosed and I was in hospital, she came to visit. We'd split up just before and I'd been staying at my Mum's . Anyway she found out I was in hospital and she came. She was beautiful. I'd forgotten how beautiful she was. We held one another; we didn't kiss, it was just a hug. But I was just blown away by her. She was my lucky charm. And she'd bought my daughter up to see me. She came and she helped me, I mean she helped me through it. Just being able to see my daughter at the time, gave me something. I mean that, it really, really helped me get well. That time I was in hospital was the first time I was diagnosed as schizophrenic. We got back together again afterwards shortly. Then we split and separated again. Then she got pregnant again. In the end we went to the doctors and said 'look is there anyway our child could be born with this mental illness.' He said 'No more than anybody else's'.

In the end she had a miscarriage at about three months. She went into hospital, I looked after my daughter, while she went into hospital. To have a DNC you know, to clean it all out. Then she fell with my son a few months later. She fell and we had my son. It was brilliant.

One of the things is that I don't want to do is to go out with a woman who has children. If I can't bring up my own children, I don't want nobody else's. I want a relationship with a woman but I don't want the baggage of children by someone else. And I don't want to get married. I wanted to marry my ex-partner.   Maybe, it might, well maybe it'll be different in time,   maybe in a year or two.

Right now I've got my two children and I see them a lot. I want to see them everyday if I can. I don't want to be living with nobody else's children because I can't bring up my own and it wouldn't be fair on them. I met a girl and we split up because I couldn't bring up her children you know.

My ex-partner said I can see the children every week but Mum says she doesn't want me to come down to stay every week. She thinks I'd be putting myself at risk for heroin and she doesn't want me to come to Bath and start using again. I don't think I would though. I got cracked, do you know what I mean? I... I don't need it. You know I see all these people that are on heroin around. I've done it man. I know what junkies look like. I've been in jail. I just don't wanna go down that road anymore and I think I've got it cracked. I've been clean for 16 months now.

I'm on methadone. The methadone is there. If I wanna use heroin, I've got methadone. I don't need to use heroin. I'm only on 28 mgs. I'm trying to bring it down so I can go on Subutex, which is a drug that if you try taking heroin on top of that, it just doesn't do it. It wouldn't give me that buzz, it doesn't pack a punch like. I could take it or leave it with heroin now. I mean it. I haven't touched it for 16 months. My ex-partner was good. I wasn't allowed to use any drugs inside the house. I wouldn't even smoke a spliff. I'd have to make it outside and smoke it outside.

Mum never helped really. I speak to my sisters more. They think that it could be...that I could have had it since I was born. The voices. Well I can remember sitting in this shed when I was younger and hearing voices like but I don't know. I've been really troubled by them. I have a lot of trouble with them. They've made me do things. Cut myself. I've ate disgusting things. I've done disgusting things. But I didn't know how to cope with it all at the time like. I mean I've drunk bleach. I've been quite tempted to, well I've wanted to stab people. I'm on Clozapine now and it's really helping me. It's really good. Sometimes I know the voices, sometimes they're the sounds of people you know, sometimes not. Sometimes they sound like people I've met. Like now I can hear your voice and I know you're not saying it but I can still hear your voice in my head saying strange things.

I'll go away now, now that I've spoken to you and I'll hear your voice talking to me. But that only goes on until something else occupies my mind like. I mean I hear voices when I'm sitting down quiet on my own and having a cigarette but when I'm talking to you the rest of them go away. But when I hear them...they know things, all the negative things I've said to you will come out. They'll have a go at me like, for telling you that I got abused. They'll have a go at me for telling you that I couldn't eat.   They're all horrible voices. I've never had a good voice.

I think the voices are society. Having a go at me for all the wrongs I've done.   Punishing me for robbing and things. Yeah, I think it's society having a go at me for all the wrongs I've done. Paying me back.

I've got the freemasons in my head too. It's very strange this but when I was in the hostel, all my friends came to visit me. I was in the room with two or three people, sitting in a chair and I'd been smoking a cigarette. All of a sudden I felt this wave go up my body and up my back. It's gone up my body and it's rolled down my arm. And my head cracked and I heard a big smack. And 'um the voices said it was, it was their way of you know,... (pauses)   sort of breaking my neck like, like some sort of hanging. You know they hang you and your neck breaks.   This was 'um the freemasons way of telling me that I was a wrong person. That I'd done wrong. Now my head always goes to the side. It was their way, instead of killing me, they got me this way. Well they did it in like Tai Chi moves. You know with certain moves they can break your neck: this was how the freemasons broke my neck. It was their way of hanging me. It's very bizarre I know. I had this wave go up my body and my head rolled down my arm and I heard a big crack. Yeah ever since then I've had to walk with my head bent down, so that I'm always reminded of it. It's really weird. It's their way of telling me that I'm wrong, that what I've done is wrong.

I tried to hang myself when I was in prison. I just had it non-stop everyday, with the voices. 'You're wrong, you're wrong' they'd go. Man every day, all the time. It was just negative voices. All the time. All the time. All the time. On the radio. I could hear them on the radio. I could hear people knocking on the window. It really screwed my head up man. I couldn't take it, I couldn't take it.

You know I stopped eating once. I was getting voices saying that if I eat a Booster, if I eat such and such, my family are gonna die because we've all gotta sit down and eat together... *(pauses)*. It's mad. We've never done that in our family. Never. Our home's really like, well my stepdad gets home first and eats, then my sister, then my brother, then my sister. I couldn't understand that, why the voices were saying we've all got to sit down and eat together . The only time we get to sit together is having Sunday lunch. I went down from 12 and a half stone to 6 and a half stone within three months. My sister saw me when she came to visit and she next time she came she bought me this big box of crisps, chocolates, drinks, lovely pies, lovely cakes.

I said 'I can't eat it'.
She said 'Don't be daft. Eat it'.

I said 'I can't'.

She said 'Why not?'.

I said 'Because I'm hearing voices telling me that the food's dirty if I eat it. I can't eat it.'

So she says 'OK. We can get round this.' She got a bit of pie and she said 'Look there's a piece of pie. You've got saliva in your mouth. The food's dirty, the foods gonna meet the saliva. It's dirty, your saliva's gonna clean it. You can eat it.'

With that I demolished the box within about half an hour.

It's very hard to explain what it's like being in prison. It's very hard to like, well getting head space in jail is hard because there's so many people in such a small space, that there's no head room for yourself. It's very horrible. I never talk about it. I really never want to go back there. I can't cope with it. I wouldn't be able to cope with another prison sentence so that's why I don't steal or nothing. It messes with my head, screws it up. I just can't cope with it.

There's drugs going round in prison. Everyone does drugs in prison and when I used to be in jail, my ex-partner used to, 'um my brother would sort my ex-partner out and she used to bring it to me. In the end I said 'Look I don't want you bringing it no-more. I'll just get it inside now.' I didn't want her to lose the children you know. Her getting into trouble just for bringing me in pot. She used to just pass it to me. She would never put it on the children though. She used to put it in my pocket and stuff. It isn't difficult you know, I've never been spotted by a screw.

I had a friend who hung himself in jail recently. Ten days ago. In Bradford. He was doing four years for robbery. I was lucky. When I hung myself in jail, I got brought round. I thought 'Thank God. Praise the Lord.' At the time I thought it was a natural thing…the right thing to do….I'm going to be no burden to anybody else when I'm dead. Society can get on without me. I felt like society revolved around me, I was being judged by it all the time. I thought well they can pick on someone else now, if I'm out of the frame. But I got brought round by the guard.

Now I do all the classes and stuff that I can. I tackled the drugs the year I was in probation. I'm trying to learn to drive. I should be able to pass in two weeks. Not the lessons but the theory. I'm skint though but I don't need to steal to get on now. I'm living in Simon House, which is like a hostel, it's a dry house, for people with drink and drug issues. It's OK. I'm not too bothered but you know I try to keep myself to myself. Obviously I've got to think about my 'er, my …not safety but I've got to think about my, you know that if I go down that road, I might have to do this or I might end up doing that. So I'm not noisy, I'm quiet really. I keep myself to myself. I don't want any bother. I go for walks. I've been trying to do to do at least three or four miles a day.

Since I've been Clozapine, I've noticed a big change in the way I hear voices and the way I deal with them. I can say 'Go away.' Or 'Go away, come back in half an hour when I'm a bit more ready.' And they'll go away and sometimes don't come back. Because in my head, I'm occupied most of the time. I'm really depressed at the moment. A bit troubled. It's just one of those things really. My mood. They wanna put me on anti-depressants but I don't want them to. It's just another addiction innit, do you know what I mean?

I went home at Easter and I'd bought my daughter presents, 'cos it was her birthday. I'd bought her a pair of trainers, really lovely they were. And I bought her a nice pair of jeans and I'd bought her ten cigarettes. I was really chuffed. Then there's this lady that comes to the hostel where I live and does hairdressing. She's like a barber, a hairdresser whatever. Anyway she says (*puts on a horrified voice*) 'Oh you bought your daughter ten cigarettes'. I said 'yeah'. And she says 'Oh you're wrong you are'. I said, 'Why?'. She told me that I shouldn't be buying my fourteen year old daughter cigarettes. I said 'look, my ex-partner lets her smoke. If she didn't smoke in the house, she'd be smoking outside. Then she'd be mixing with all these people

269

who are out smoking behind their mum's back.' She really had a go at me, this woman, and it's really twisted my head. 'Cos I thought yeah, but she'll start stealing money to buy cigarettes. I said if we didn't give her cigarettes, she'd be stealing money for cigarettes. Then she'll be hanging around with all the wrong people because they smoke. And they'll drink. It really twisted my head that did and that didn't help. I've been thinking about it a lot. It's messed my head up. So...so when I go to see them next time, next month, I'm gonna pull my ex-partner up and say look I'm not trying to have a go at Kylie but I'd appreciate it if, I'd appreciate it, if you don't mind me not getting her cigarettes anymore.

I worry about my kids taking drugs. Hopefully you know, they've got a good stable background. They've never really been brought up with drugs around them. My daughter says no, she'll never do them. My son, I don't think he'll ever do them. I think he's gonna go into the army. Obviously 'cos of, with his stepdad and everything. So I think my son might go that way. Which I'm grateful for. I hope he does. I mean I would rather have done ten years in the army than ten years in jail. You get paid for it man. I mean you go round the world, all exotic places. I mean I know you go to war sometimes, and you gotta be peacekeepers and things like that, but I think it would be a good career, a good life for my son. But then again he could join the Peace Corps or something like that if he wants to.

I'm happy whatever he chooses. I'd like to help him as much as I can.

I'm hoping for my mental health to get better and better and for my relationship with my mum and my family to get better. I'm hoping to see my children as much as I can. I just hope for a better quality of life now I'm on Clozapine and I think I've got my drug addiction under control. I've done 16 months but I think I've got it cracked now, you know. I go to a drugs drop-in-centre regularly. I go to a drugs counsellor at my GP and I see a drugs worker that comes to the hostel. I do try to occupy my time as much as possible. I mean I'd like to do, not a job but a night course or something like that. I have problems at night. I hear voices sometimes until I sleep. It's not just that though, I mean I could be doing something better with my life if I did a course or something. Even if it's just for two hours a night. At least it'd be something constructive. Instead of sitting and watching 'EastEnders' and stuff like that, I'd be out like learning how to use a computer, *(pauses)*... or doing an English course. I'm not very good at English or Maths but basic, basic I can do. I need help the more I do it though, it's very hard for me to learn now. It might get easier. But hopefully it's something I could do.

I'm hoping to be happy and I think I deserve to be happy now. That's what I want really.

A Carer's Perspective; Edward

Joy's son Edward committed suicide in 2002. I was incredibly nervous before meeting Joy because I knew the story she had to tell was such a sad one. However, as soon as I met her, Joy emanated warmth and this was the same each following time we met. A couple of months after giving this interview Joy retired. She is currently in the process of taking legal action against the Mental Health Trust who were responsible for Edward when he died.

Edward was different to his brother and sister. He was different even as a baby. He was so physically strong, he was pulling himself up in the cot at six months and walking at nine months. He did more damage to the things in the house than the other two put together because he didn't understand the word 'no'. When the other two started walking they knew what 'no' meant, so if they went near anything, you'd just say 'no' whereas he just carried on. So things did get broken and we realised we had to start moving things up whereas we taught the others to respect people's things. You couldn't do that with a nine month old baby *(laughs)*. And that's the way Edward carried on really. *(laughs)*

He was...he was a sweet little thing – always talking, always chatting. Very active. He used to have lots and lots of energy. I remember talking to his infant teacher after he died, she lived in the village at that point, strange enough. She contacted me with some photos of him when he was at school, and asked me round for coffee. She said what she remembers of Edward more than anything was the fact that though he was quite mischievous, he was also very interested in anything that was going on in class. He was one of those who always had his hand up, wanting to be involved. Whatever they were doing, he wanted to be part of it. And that was Edward. He always wanted to know what was happening, why it was happening.

Memories of him as a child are of a very cheerful, happy little boy. He wasn't....he wasn't one...well he liked books and when he was older he read books and he liked having books read to him and though he was very artistic and he enjoyed drawing, he was somebody who needed a lot of physical activity. He had loads of energy that needed to be burnt off to get him to sleep.

He did get into a lot of mischief, he got into all sorts of things. He got chased around the village once by one of his friend's fathers. Him and another friend had picked up some bricks that someone had piled up neatly by the brook. There was a stream in our old village and someone had piled some bricks neatly at the bottom of their garden and the boys had come along and thrown them in the brook. The man had come out and caught them and he chased them all round the village. They came back in - Matthew was staying for tea - and I knew there was something wrong because of their expressions. They'd said they weren't hungry and they went rushing upstairs to the bedroom.   I went up after them and asked them what was wrong and eventually Edward said that they'd thrown some bricks they'd found at the end of Mr Kirby's garden and he'd chased them all round the village.

'But I don't think he knows it was us,' he said, 'we went up the footpath and we hid and he couldn't find us.'

So I said, 'Well what are you going to do?'

He said 'Do you think he'll call the police?'

I said – they were only about 6 or 7 at this stage – and I said that I really didn't know what he was going to do but I could tell them what they could do. They both sat wide eyed looking at me and I said that if they went up to Mr Kirby's and knocked on the door and apologised for what they'd done, that they'd probably feel better and feel like having their tea. They looked at each other obviously not wanting to do this. I said I'd go with them. So eventually and very reluctantly, they decided that was probably the best course of action.

We went up to Mr Kirby's and actually David was trying very hard not to laugh as they were apologising and saying what they'd done. He explained to them that he'd spent all Sunday afternoon piling the bricks up and it would be very helpful if they'd go and pick the bricks up out of the brook and put them back on the ground. They went and did that and they came back and had their tea and realised that that was …well, a much simpler thing to do than spending their time worrying about it. I think in a way that experience made Edward quite open and truthful, it was almost like, whenever he did anything, if he dropped something, or broke something he wasn't like the other two who tried to hide it first and then admit to it. He used to just come in and say 'Mum, I've done so and so'. So I think perhaps that that was a lesson which it was worth him learning; that it was easier to own up and when he did he found it wasn't quite so bad. I think also when he did tell lies…'um I could read them with him - until he got older - but when he was young I always knew when he was lying. He couldn't look at you directly and his face went red and there was a slight sort of look about him that you knew whatever it was wasn't true and he'd eventually have to tell you the truth.

He was very good at Maths, very clever at Maths. And quite musical…I've read somewhere that Maths and Music actually go together. He could pick out tunes. He'd hear a tune in his head and he could go and play it on the piano. He passed a common entrance exam to a Prep. School when we were thinking about moving him from the village school. At the time in the village school, there were only boys in the class - well there were nine boys in his class who were all older than him and there were about three boys in the lower class – there were only two classes in the school – and they were younger than him. Of course he mixed with the older ones which for someone like Edward who was bright enough and got himself into enough trouble, well, he didn't exactly need the help of the older ones. We knew we'd have to change schools because we wanted him to mix with children of his own age. We thought it would be better for him. We were going to go for the school in the next village, it was only the fact that we saw the Prep. School had a common entry exam that we went along to see if he was any good and he actually passed it. He was accepted into the school and we decided that as the other two were quite a bit older, we could probably afford to pay for him to go to this school…so that's where he went.

He was quite angry at first, he didn't want to go. When we went to…they had a sort of classroom where they used to have second hand uniforms, and I took him along there to buy the uniform. The whole time he was there he was going around saying I don't know why you're buying this because I'm not coming to this school. It was really embarrassing with all these other parents there *(laughs)*. I mean some were just like us, just ordinary but there were some quite, sort of, well-to-do people there. There was me with this awkward child who didn't want to try anything on and was insisting quite loudly that he wasn't going to try anything on. It was quite an embarrassing experience.

He started the school though and after the first term he actually enjoyed it. He discovered that they played sport every afternoon which got rid of all the pent up energy he had. He also found that he could do music and he learnt...he started to learn the clarinet. He had really wanted to play the saxophone but he needed to learn the clarinet first and he started to learn to read music. They also had a very good art department and he started learning how to draw and things. The art teacher – when I spoke to him again after Edward died - said he had recognised Edward's talent and that he'd had talent beyond his years. He was in fact, like a mentor to Edward and encouraged him and showed him all sorts of different mediums and things and Edward learnt a lot of skills from him because he recognised what Edward had.

When he got to ten he suddenly decided he wanted to board. I wasn't happy and didn't want him to because I was totally anti-boarding school. But it was only weekdays and he came home at weekends. The reason he wanted to board was because all his friends were. He could get up early in the morning and they had a swimming pool where they went swimming in the summer. They used to have raids in and out of each other's dormitories and things *(laughs)* and so...His head teacher or the boarding house teacher or whatever the right name was, was the art teacher and he lived there with his wife and he had two little children. In the evenings, he used to ask a chosen few – and Edward happened to be one of them, one of the arty ones - to go down and have toast and hot chocolate in his sitting room before they went to bed. *(laughs)*

I think, you know, he was, he was very, very happy at that school. It showed in all his work and his outlook in life and though he left that school when he was twelve, nearly thirteen, all the friends that he made there turned up at his funeral and that was when you know, he was twenty. They still kept in touch and when one of them heard they just let everybody else know. Most of the teachers that weren't teaching at that time came to the funeral as well, so all in all it was a very special school. It was somewhere where I knew Edward was happy... *(pauses)*

When he was fifteen, I took out a loan – his father and I went through a divorce when Edward was between the ages of fourteen and fifteen. It wasn't an easy thing, it was very difficult... My ex-husband, Ed's father, couldn't take what was happening and he was... he caused quite a lot of problems. I decided that Edward needed a good holiday. I talked to a friend, another mother who had her son at the school; in fact her son, Henry, was Edward's best friend. She had just come through a divorce as well - and she wanted to take Henry away and we decided to take them to

Disneyworld. I took out a loan which was...well, it was quite an expensive holiday, but it was the last holiday I ever had with Edward. I don't regret a penny of it because we had a really, really good time and Edward was still Edward at that point. It's something that I'll treasure because I've still got the photographs. I just know, I know he was happy there. We were all happy and we had a great time. That's something I'll never regret.

It was not long after that, that I noticed things weren't quite right with Edward. I discovered shortly after we came back that he was smoking because I smelt cigarette smoke on him and noticed the stains on his fingers. I didn't know at that time that he was involved in cannabis, I just knew he was smoking. He'd left the Prep. school – he'd actually passed an Arts scholarship – and had gone onto another (private) school and 'um...he wasn't happy there. He got mixed up in the wrong crowd and part of his escape was smoking cannabis. But you know, I was a child of the Sixties, I didn't see that much harm in it. I didn't really think it could do any damage. I don't know - when I say it was his escape - I don't know if at that stage if he was beginning to hear voices or experience delusions, and cannabis was a way of escaping. Or if cannabis triggered what happened to him later. I just don't know. But I feel it's all tied in somewhere with the general unhappiness he seemed to be experiencing and everything.

He got picked for the 'A' team in rugby but soon after he did his ankle in and he was out for the season. He'd got a try. His first try with the school, you know, and everybody was, you know, buoying him up saying 'well done' and everything. Then the next session he did something to his ankle; he tore all his tendons and things in it and he was out for the rest of the rugby season. He wasn't able to play football either. And when he tried to do rowing his ankle swelled up again, so he didn't, he couldn't go into rowing. So the sports side, which I think could have saved him, didn't really take off. But he was..., he had been a good rugby player ....he played for the 'A' team all the way through when he was at Prep-school. He used to go skiing there as well and he got a medal for skiing, a bronze medal. And he got a gold medal for judo in the inter-school championships. We used to have to sit there for hours *(laughs)*. It was quite boring watching all these lads. I mean it was a Sunday wasted to me. There used to be heats and because he was good they would start at half past eight and we wouldn't get away until half past five. All you could get was a hot dog and a horrible tasting coffee *(laughs)*. I used to have to remember to take sandwiches. It wasn't a good experience for us, but Edward obviously enjoyed it. It was a good experience for him. He was quite proud of it all. They did take a photograph, which I haven't got unfortunately. The school got one with him and the team holding the cup, and because Edward had got the medal he was holding the cup. So that was good.

Yes, things started going wrong when he got to fifteen, sixteen. It's difficult to explain why, or what caused it... *(pauses)* First of all, he started... he started cutting off his friends. It went from having a house full of friends or, or from someone always ferrying him – well not me because I didn't drive – but his sister or his dad ferrying him somewhere and then having to pick him up a day later because he was staying out, to nothing. He started refusing to speak to people on the phone. Not asking them round anymore and just saying 'oh I'm not friends with them anymore'. I never knew why and he could never explain why. He'd just say 'Oh, oh, we're just not friends anymore. He's stupid.' Things like that. I found that hard to understand. Then he started to put things up against the bedroom door and locking his bedroom door. He began to have a thing about me making sure the front door was locked before we went to bed. This was during the time when we'd moved to a new house. The divorce had gone through and the old house had been sold. At this time there was just me and Emma and Edward there. James had been with us for a while, but then he saved up and managed to get a place with his girlfriend. So it was the three of us who were in that house and he had this thing about making sure everything was locked up and sometimes getting up and

281

checking. When I went into his room in the morning to call him for school, I'd have to push things away from the door to get in. He started accusing me of going into his room and searching for things. Interfering and spying on him. None of it was true of course, but for him it was happening and you just couldn't explain to him that we weren't doing anything. Sometimes he'd get so angry with me he'd go over and stay with his dad. The awkward thing there was, Richard hadn't accepted that we were divorced and he was harassing me quite a bit. The police were involved. He wasn't allowed to come near the house and things. That was hard. That was hard on everybody... *(pauses)*

Richard was also saying to Edward at that time, that he was going to kill himself if I didn't have him back. I mean Edward was only sixteen and I got really angry. I can remember asking him – Richard - to actually come round and trying to tell him that he was putting an awful lot onto someone of that age. That it was difficult enough growing up and that Edward was facing enough emotional things without having to deal with that. Edward had come home one evening crying and saying 'Dad keeps saying he's gonna kill himself Mum and I don't know what to do'. I tried to say, well, that maybe he shouldn't see his dad for a while. To get a bit of space. And he said 'No, I need to see him, he's got no-one else.' He'd started feeling responsible for his dad and I did feel that was difficult for him. They seemed to get over it though. Then they seemed to go through a phase where they were arguing an awful lot and Edward would go down and see him and the next thing was he'd be ringing up asking to be collected.

I don't really know what they were arguing about. Richard can be a very difficult man. Sometimes he used to say things and then deny he'd said them. And that used, that's what caused trouble between him and I. Edward, at that point, was a very astute person and it was just..., *(pauses)* I don't know...things were difficult. He used to come back and he used to tell me about it and I used to say 'Well you know that's what dad's like'. But he used to be angry, very angry with him.

He started at a local college of further education. He'd told me just before he was about to take his GCSEs' that he hated the school he was at and he wanted to leave. I eventually managed to persuade him to stay and he sat his exams and did reasonably well. He got 8 GCSEs'; all quite good results, in fact he got an A Star for Art. Anyway he wanted to go on to college, to take his art. He wanted to take art, an 'A' level in art, media studies and .... I think it was sociology he was thinking of doing. He went for the interview and he was accepted and everything seemed fine when he started in the September. He seemed quite happy there at the beginning. He went off on the bus every day and things. He met a girl there and got himself handcuffed to her somehow or other. It was some sort of joke - his mates handcuffed them you know. I think he was interested in her and she was interested in him, but they couldn't get it together so mates put in a helping hand *(laughs)*. She came round a few times. Edward had a fit of giggles when she stayed for a meal because he wasn't used to this sort of thing *(laughs)*. Then they fell out, for what reason or how or what happened, I don't know. It suddenly just seem to end. I think he was quite upset but he never said very much about it.

He decided he wanted to change from sociology to psychology and then changed his mind again. Then he decided he'd been better off before and wanted to change back. Obviously by then the teachers were getting annoyed with him. He also had some problems with the art teacher. I never met her but sometimes he used to come back very upset by her. He was doing graphics at the time, something which he hadn't done before. And she kept saying to him was 'You're an A star student. I haven't seen any A star work yet'. I think she really, really knocked his confidence. I think he lost a lot of confidence and self-esteem through this teacher because art was one thing that he felt confident in and with, and thought he was good at. I think this, that this criticism didn't do him any good.

I can remember going up and speaking to someone on an open day. I didn't see the actual art teacher, but I spoke to the teacher who was in charge, his sort of, form teacher or whatever, and said I wasn't happy. I said, you know, he may be, well he was very good at fine art, but that doesn't mean he's good at every other kind of art. When he went in again after the half term, he started to do figure drawing and they noticed that he was very quick at getting the shapes down and he didn't have to redo it. He could just look and do it. So that particular teacher understood, you know, that he did have talent but the one that was doing the graphics was someone else.

Then just before he was due to go back after Christmas, I got a letter from the college, asking me whether he was going to return in January. I said to Edward 'What's this? It says you haven't been there for a few weeks in December. They want to know if you're going back'. So he said, 'Well of course I'm going back'. I asked him why hadn't he been going and he said he'd been going to this sort of, this drop in centre, or something in town. He said that he just sat there and smoked until it was time to go home again. He couldn't tell me why and I just couldn't understand. I really didn't understand what was going on. Anyway I had to go and see the Head to explain why Edward, well basically that Edward was coming back. On the day of the appointment, Edward decided he was too ill to come and that he had flu. He obviously didn't want to go with me, so I had to go on my own. I went and I apologised on his behalf and I explained about the fact that Edward's father and I hadn't long been divorced and that there were still some problems with him. There were still things going on Edward and Richard at this time. Anyway I said that he was definitely going to attend this term because Edward assured me that he really did want to come back.

The long and short of it was, he went back but he didn't even stick it out until the half term. He came home one night very down and said he didn't want to go to college anymore. I explained to him that if he was giving up college, that was fine, he didn't have to stay if that wasn't what he wanted to do, but that I was struggling to pay the mortgage and take care of him and the house and all the expenses. I told him that he would need to get a job. He agreed but said he needed a couple of weeks off. I didn't mind that but I did tell him that he really needed to start looking for some work because I just couldn't afford to take care of him. And he never, ever did get a job. He started staying awake most of the night and sleeping during the day. I used to get home from work and he would have just got up and he'd just be making himself some egg and bacon for breakfast. It was .... it was horrible .... I couldn't talk to him. He would go up into his room and shut himself in. There was just no communication.

Then at one point during the summer - what would have been the summer holidays if he'd have been at college - I had a couple of days off and I was sitting at home and he was sitting down as well and he suddenly started talking and was quite communicative. He told me that a while a go he'd had a phone call from one of his friends offering him some cocaine or something and Edward said he'd gone round and that they'd spiked his drink. That he'd been aware of things going on but that he couldn't stop them and that he'd been gang-raped.

Obviously I was totally shocked and didn't know what to say. I asked him when it had happened and he said not long after Christmas, after he'd gone back to college. So it was seemed a long time ago. I said, 'Why didn't you tell me then?' and we had... we had a long talk about it. In the end, I just said 'Edward, I think we both need a hug'. And we got up and I hugged him, I mean I was almost in tears. I didn't know how to handle it or what to do. Except that I did say that I think he needed to have an Aids test. I talked it over with Nigel (my new partner), who I'd met around the same year. Edward hadn't wanted anyone to know but I said that I needed to talk to somebody and did he mind if I talked to Nigel? And he had.... He did like Nigel. He had a lot of respect for Nigel. Nigel sort of said, that he'd come with us.

So we did take him for an Aids test. And he was okay. They actually, they talked to him, counselled him when he went there. He was in there quite a while. But we didn't do anything else about it because we didn't know what to do. There was no point going to the police because it was too late. And he couldn't remember it all properly....he changed his story halfway through about how this stuff was given to him, he thought it was something called Ketamine or something like that. He said he kept having terrible flashbacks and things, but now I don't really know whether that was a delusion. It was possibly his first delusion and at the time it seemed real. I don't know, it may all be tied together. Or maybe this incident triggered the schizophrenia and it really did happen.

He then decided he wanted to go back to college and I had a hell of a job trying to get him back in. He wanted to do Btec art and I had to really plead and promise that he would go back. That he would behave and work and go in. I knew the guy who was the caretaker there and he knew some of the people who worked there and he spoke to the Head. In the end they agreed and they accepted him but he had to get a portfolio together, which was very difficult. He did actually sit down and do some drawings. I'd said that if he really, really honestly did want to go back, then to start doing some drawings and let me see some proof, because that's what the school wanted. And he did.

The boys he accused of gang raping him were in the second year by then. He'd had to start at the bottom again. He then started saying that....I can't remember the boy's name, it was Danny or something, was sticking a needle into Edward's leg every time he walked past and injecting him. I said 'Edward, I don't think so'. And he swore, he swore that it was happening. He said he could feel it go in every time this boy passed him. He accused his dad of doing the same thing a year or so later as well.

Anyway it came to his 18th birthday. He went to college in the day and in the evening we were having a family dinner. When he came back we were going to give him his presents and things. We'd....there was a special watch he wanted which was about £200 and I couldn't afford it, but all the family together bought it because we thought, 'Well, it's his 18th. It's special.' So we'd clubbed together and got him this watch. That was going to be presented to him. And he came back stoned. It was obvious he'd been smoking Cannabis. I mean you could tell by his eyes. 'Oh, it's my birthday' he said. He managed to sort himself out and behave himself though. We gave him his watch and everything seemed alright, but the next morning he got up and he just announced that he wasn't going to go to college anymore. Yes, the day after his 18th birthday he announced

'I don't want to go to college anymore, I want to go and live in London'.

I was totally shocked, this seemed completely out of the blue. I wanted to know why and he said 'Nothing here holds anything for me anymore. There's nothing here for me. I want to go and live in London. I want to go to Art College in London'. I asked him how he was going to finance it all. He said that he'd get a job in McDonalds and save and go to college. He wanted to go to Camberwell Art College. And I said 'Well you haven't actually got the qualifications yet. You've got to have your A levels and things'. He said he was going to go and do them at evening classes. I mean he'd obviously thought it out. I used to take him to London a lot when he was younger. Him and his friend Henry. We did The Tower of London and Madame Tussaud's and various things. We also went to places like Camden Lock and Covent Garden. All of which he loved, so you know, I think he found that after being brought up in a very quiet, tiny village of about six hundred people, that London was really buzzing.

Of course I tried to persuade him to stay and I offered him places in….well I said I'd find somewhere in Oxford, find somewhere in Reading, in Didcot. By then Nigel and I were looking for a house, we'd decided we were going to live together. Edward was quite pleased about it. Emma was living with us then, but she said she wanted to get a place of her own, so she got a place. We were quite flexible about where we were going to live and eventually we found this place here. Edward liked it and he knew some people in the village. There's a little room at the back of the house and he'd already asked if he could he have that as his room, where he could play his music and have his friends round. This was when….well what friends, I don't know because he didn't actually see anyone at the time. At least he was thinking about the future and it seemed positive and I thought well, you know ok and we said yes. Yes, that it could be his room. Everything seemed to be alright.

So this thing about London came as a bit of a shock. I can remember saying to him, 'Well, I realise maybe you don't want to live with us. That's understandable and you don't have to come and live with us. You're 18. But I don't really want you living so far away'. I offered him an old car and driving lessons so that he could get around. Nothing worked….he was absolutely determined to go to London and if he didn't get any help, he was just going to pack up and go. In the end, I'd sold my house and Nigel had sold his and we were moving into this one and I had some savings. I financed his move and I paid 3 months rent in London, which was extremely expensive and also put £3000 in a bank account for him. I arranged for him to have an appointment at the job centre or whatever was around for the youth of that time, I can't remember exactly. Anyway we went and met the right people and they told him that as soon as he'd moved he should go and see them and they'd help sort him out. Get him signed on and things. We also went down the college and various things, to all the local places. He moved two days after we moved in here.

Richard helped him move because we were also moving Emma in as well. In the end he was there for 3 months and I actually never, ever got to see the inside of the flat. We went up there once and we couldn't get him to answer the door. I think he was in, the curtains were pulled, his mobile phone was in there because we could hear it ringing, and he never ever went anywhere without his mobile phone. We spent an hour and a half trying to get in and I ended up pushing a very angry note under his door and coming home. He'd asked for a plant and we'd left the plant outside the door. He'd said he'd wanted a new plant for his flat. Then after 3 months he suddenly came home... we don't know, well we don't know why. He left the flat for two weeks before he even told us, he...he lived in a horrible place in Paddington, near Paddington Station. It must have been - I don't know - a hostel or something. I'm not really sure. I just know it was awful because he said that the toilets and the bathroom were so dirty he used to go down to Paddington Station to use the washing facilities and things. As far as I know he stayed there for two weeks.

Within that time he stole some traveller's cheques. I didn't know about this at the time, I only found out later. Apparently he tried to cash them in, in Oxford, and got caught. They traced him to Richard's, where he was staying. He must have been arrested, I don't know. Afterwards he came home here. He told me he had to go to court in Hammersmith, and it was because he'd been caught in a fight. Nigel and I couldn't work out exactly what was going on. I knew he was lying or that the whole truth wasn't coming out. He'd said that he was with three friends and that he was the one that was having to go to court. I wanted to know why the others weren't going and why....why the other people were suing him or taking him to court when, well, if it was a fight, there were two sides. You just couldn't get the full story out of him.

I wanted to go to court with him and he was extremely angry about it and said he didn't want me there. We argued a lot about it. He was totally adamant that he didn't want me there. Around that time he'd been talking to a girl on the Internet. He told me he was in love with somebody he'd met on the Internet. They met up and they got on very well. I met her, she came and stayed here a few times. Her name was Kirsty. She was a really lovely girl. She was the same age as Edward but *(laughs)* a hell of a lot older than Edward. Edward, though he was 18, getting on for 19, was more like a 15 year old. Still very dependent on me for doing a lot of things for him. Kirsty was very grown up. She had a job and was encouraging Edward to get a job. And to do things. Encouraging him to do his A-levels so he could go to Art College. She was Edward's first love really, his only love as it turned out.

Anyway she went to court with him and they came back here afterwards and she sort of said, 'It's alright, everything's ok. I'll look after him, I'll keep an eye on him' and I believed her because she was, she was just lovely. Edward was besotted with her. She came from Tunbridge Wells, and as it's quite a long way from here to Tunbridge Wells. He decided he wanted to go back to London again because it was halfway. He said it was easier for Kirsty to come and visit him and for him to visit her and I understood that. I still didn't want him to go back and by this time he'd also been given a bond by the local housing association. He would have had a flat to live in if he'd stayed here.

He decided not to use it and go back to London. He was looking up hostels on the Internet. I really, really didn't want him to go to a hostel, I explained to him that he was only allowed there for a little while and that he'd have to move on. That he couldn't stay there forever. I said I was worried that he'd end up homeless. Eventually the last of my savings went on getting another flat for Edward so that he and Kirsty could be together....well.... Within a couple of months – I think he must have gone back to London in the July and in what would have been about the beginning of September - they broke up. He was very jealous of her. Not of her but about her. He was so jealous and I kept trying to explain to him that you need, you really needed trust in a relationship. I said that if you love somebody you trust them. She worked in a shop, a grocery store and the hours were different. Sometimes they didn't close till ten o'clock and Edward wouldn't accept that shops were still open at ten o'clock. I was saying well yes, sometimes they were. He was convinced that she was going off and meeting other boys. We had lots of talks on trust and that and he'd say 'Yeah, yeah, you're right', but he couldn't accept it. I think that he wasn't....well basically he wasn't well. They broke up and he became very, very, very depressed, very unhappy. He was binge drinking or drinking quite heavily anyway. Even when he came back here, he would drink. I ended up locking away any alcohol we had, locking it in the shed. He was drinking so heavily it worried me.

Then his 19th birthday arrived. Was it his 19th? Let me think. Yes his 19th birthday, in the November. He came back home and we had a sort of dinner. I always... I have this thing that I'll always cook a meal for the family, for whoever's birthday it is. If I don't take them out for a meal, we'll still have a meal and we'll all get together. When he came over though he was very, very down. He was so down and he just sat with his head dropped down the whole time. He seemed so very unhappy that I didn't actually want him to go back. But he wanted to and when his brother left, Edward asked him to drop him off at the station. I said 'Why don't you stay the night?', but he was adamant he wanted to go back to London.

I phoned every day that week and I couldn't get hold of him and was really worried. By the weekend, I wanted to go up there and find out what had happened because I just couldn't get any reply. It wasn't just once a day, I phoned several times. While I was at work, when I came home and in the evenings. I kept thinking that eventually he must answer the phone. In the end I rang Richard, his father, and I asked him if he'd heard anything from Edward and he said 'Oh, he's here'. He said there had been a fire in his flat and all his stuff had been destroyed. He'd phoned Richard up and asked him to come and get him. I said, 'well I wish you'd told me, I've been worrying all week'. We found out quite a bit later while Edward was in hospital that Edward had actually started the fire. He was seemed to have been hallucinating at the time. He talked to his psychiatrist about it when he was in hospital. But at the time we knew nothing about it, how it started or anything.

He came to see me and he said that he still wanted to go back to London. At the time my sister and brother-in-law were here and they offered to take him back to Hertfordshire, because they had a place there. Well, they lived there and Hertfordshire was closer to London than here and it would be easier for him to get in.

So he went back to stay with them. He was there for a couple of weeks. Simon, my brother-in-law was actually getting him up and taking him into work with him. He had a delivery job delivering paint and things and he was taking Edward and getting him to deliver. And ....the only problem was that Simon was a born again Christian. He called himself a pastor. He used to hold Sunday....things, meetings in his house. I think Edward got involved and....I don't know....I don't know the full story of what happened. I know that he put his hand on Edward's head to give him the power and everything. To take away all the evil things. I think this really affected Edward quite badly. I noticed Edward became quite loving on the phone when you spoke to him, in a way that was unusual for him.

One weekend I was going up to Cromer to see my brother just before Christmas. Edward had phoned up and said he was coming home. Simon and Sue were coming down to visit some friends nearby and they were going to drop Edward off here. I explained that I would be at my brothers seeing them and giving them their presents. He seemed ok and said that he'd go and see his dad. Richard told me that when Edward arrived he hugged him and said 'Dad, I love you. It's good to see you' and all this sort of stuff. Richard said he was completely different to how he'd ever seen him before. He was also, he said, very strange; they went to watch the local football team play and when they came back and Edward said 'They're going to win the cup final, I've willed them. I can do it with my brain now and they will be able to win the cup final'....*(pauses)* He ...he was kind of preaching to Richard about God and things. He kept talking about Danny Damiola, the young boy that had died and that he had, that he had the power to bring him back to life. That he knew how to do it. Anyway Richard and him had some sort of argument - I don't know what it was about - but Edward walked out. Richard said it was pouring with rain and Edward had no coat, no money. He wasn't dressed for the weather; the pouring rain in December.

He phoned Richard at about quarter to four in the morning to ask him to come and pick him up and he was quite near here. Whether he was trying to get to here and then suddenly remembered I wasn't there and then walked on, I don't know, but Richard collected him. He said he was in a terrible mess, covered in mud, soaking wet and speaking a lot of nonsense. Said he'd met some ghosts and things. Richard cleaned him up, washed him and put him to bed.

The next morning Richard told him he was going to his grandmother's for lunch and when they got there, Edward got out of the car and said 'I'm not going in, I want to go back to Hertfordshire'. Richard explained that Simon and Sue would pick him up later. But Edward said 'No, I'm going now, take me to the station'. Richard refused and Edward walked off again and he disappeared for 36 hours.

Simon and Sue had rung me in Cromer and asked where Edward was because they were supposed to be taking him back. I didn't know what was going on. When we got back, I heard from Richard the story of what had gone on ....I couldn't understand why he hadn't done anything. The following morning I went to the police and took a photograph of Edward. I explained what had happened and I said that I felt that his thoughts were very irrational and that I was worried about his mental health. The police agreed and said that they'd put the photograph out and do their best to try and find him. Eventually he was picked up in Stevenage outside the cinema, watching a woman in the kiosk. Simon had said that the week before they'd gone to the cinema and he'd fallen hopelessly in love with the girl who worked there. He'd called her an angel and he'd drawn a picture of her - Simon said it looked just like her – when he'd got back home. He was picked up while he standing outside the cinema watching her or waiting for her, we presume. The police took him back and they put him into Simon and Sue's custody, for them to look after him.

Simon rang me sometime later and he said 'Joy, we're bringing Edward home, we think he's very ill and he needs to see a doctor'.

I said 'Ok, I'll let the doctor know.' I rang my GP and explained to him what was happening. In the meantime, Simon then rang back and said 'We're having trouble, Edward won't leave the house and he's getting quite irate and we're not sure what to do'. I asked to speak to him. And Edward was very sharp and said 'I'll be back but I'm not going to come back yet. I'll be back….on Friday. I'll see you on Friday night'.

It was Monday. I said 'yes, yes, ok, fine'.

He said 'And Simon's trying to make me sit down, I don't want to sit down'.

I said 'It's ok, you don't have to sit down. Give me Simon again'.

I spoke to Simon and I just explained to him that I felt he needed to leave Edward alone and let him calm down. And I said 'Don't try to make him do something he doesn't want to do. If he wants to stand up, let him stand' sort of thing. I also asked him to get Sue to ring me from her mobile outside. When she rang me, I just said 'Sue, I'm really scared and worried about Edward and I give you permission to phone the police because I think he does need to see a doctor and I think calling the police is the only way to do it.' I said 'Don't feel bad about it. I give you permission to do it'. So that's what they did. When the police arrived Edward was calm and he was sitting down and he spoke to this policeman ordinarily in a way, I mean very calmly, telling him that he was in touch with the Pope and that he was the Son of God and that he was collecting up all the evil spirits in the world and that he was going to make the world a better place for everybody. The other policeman who was with him, went into Sue's kitchen and was speaking to the Sergeant or whoever at the station and was saying that it was the strangest case he'd ever seen. That Edward was certainly irrational and certainly mentally ill but that he was so calm with it, that he – the policeman - he'd never seen anything like it. Whoever was at the station said that they needed to get him to the hospital. They went back and said to Edward that they thought he needed to see a doctor and he just said if that what they thought and they were the police, they must be right, then that was what he needed to do. He went outside and unfortunately there they handcuffed him - I don't know why because he was calm and complying with everything they said - and put him into a police car and he was taken to a nearby hospital.

The ward for the mentally sick where he was taken was right at the top of the building. I'm not sure what floor, but high up and it was a locked ward. Edward was in a little room with a tiny window in it and he - delusional at the time anyway - thought he was in prison. I went to see him the next day and he burst into tears and I just held him. He kept saying 'Why am I in here? I've done nothing wrong Mum, why are they locking me up? Why am I in here?' I kept trying to explain to him that we knew he hadn't done anything wrong and that he was ill, but he couldn't accept it. He felt that the Government and everybody were against him. As I said he had a thing about God by then. He was very, very religious. He'd drawn a cross and put it up on the wall. It was a miserable little room anyway. He had an old Bible he'd found in a drawer in the ward and he was reading that to me. When I related it to Nigel later I said it was like the sermon on the windowsill, because he sat up there and he was spouting out all this stuff. Reading bits from the Bible and then explaining to me what he thought it all meant. Later on he wanted a sandwich and he wasn't allowed to leave the ward so that caused a problem and he got upset. As well as a sandwich, he wanted a Bible. He was very insistent on the Bible. However there was nowhere I could have bought a Bible at that time and when I went back with the sandwich and the drink, he got quite angry. That's when I really cried. He was so unlike Edward and so unlike anyone I'd ever seen before or dealt with....I didn't know how to handle it.

I was asked to go into this room with a long table and people sitting round the whole of the table and they all introduced themselves. There were art therapists, drama therapists, trainee this and trainee that. There were so many people. The consultant spoke to me and he just said 'We think your son is very, very close to schizophrenia and he needs medication straight away'. I asked them to start it, to do whatever they needed to do, to help him. Then up came the thing that he wasn't a resident of that area and that he lived in another county and that he needed to be moved back there. He didn't actually get treated while he was there. He stayed for a week while they found somewhere to transfer him, but he never had any real treatment. He was just sectioned so he couldn't leave the ward.

When he was eventually transferred, they started the assessment thing and were trying to give him medication. At the time he wouldn't take it properly. I used to go in to visit and he'd show it to me. He would have it in his hand and I used to report it when I went out, that he wasn't taking it, that he still had it on him. They'd stay and watch him take it but I think he still held it in his mouth and then spat it out afterwards. He knew what to do, yes he knew what to do. He was....he was incredibly ill at that time and so delusional. He really believed he was God, or the Son of God or whatever. He was very strange and he'd say, sometimes he'd say quite horrible things.

For Christmas he demanded a white tracksuit which proved was absolutely impossible to find. I got him a light grey one but he gave it to the nurse in the end and told her to give them to Oxfam. I used to take him in fruit and things and he'd squash all that into the bin. He wanted tapes and then he pulled all the tapes apart. Everything you gave him, everything you did, he destroyed. He wanted some Nike trainers, white with a gold tick on the side, to go with the tracksuit so he could look like the Son of God. He gave those to the nurses for Oxfam. Of course the nurses just gave them to me, and I gave to them to him again later when he got a bit better.

While he was staying there he was pushing things up against the door again, saying he was being raped. That the food was poisoned. He wouldn't eat the food. He was...it was horrific actually. We went to see him on Christmas Day and he said to James, his brother, he said 'I don't care about any of you, none of you mean anything to me. My family could walk out and get run over by a bus tomorrow and I wouldn't care. It wouldn't affect me at all. I just don't care about any of you'. James really took it to heart and really believed it and it took a long time for me to convince James that, well that it wasn't Edward talking. It was the illness and that Edward would never, ever have said anything like that. I was trying to get him to see through the illness and to say that underneath there was a very frightened person....who needed to know that he was loved, even though he didn't seem like himself. That somewhere in there, there was a person who needed to know that we still cared about him. That we weren't going to turn against him because he was so strange. James couldn't accept it though and he stayed away for a long time, wouldn't visit him.

I visited everyday. I didn't miss a day. Then after Christmas an awful thing happened. He was due for a mental health tribunal because he was appealing against the sectioning. God, it was supposed to be happening just after Christmas, well, after the New Year. Then they decided to do it on the 29th of December and on the 28th December I got a phone call to say it was going ahead the next day. I arrived on the 29th; Edward's father couldn't come because he was down in Wales and it had been snowing so he couldn't travel down in time. Edward's CPN couldn't be there, so somebody was standing in. Edward's solicitor, who had seen him and who'd spoken to me and had said 'Your son's really ill'. You see the first time she saw him, she thought he was ok. She'd only seen him briefly and he had managed to keep up an act. So originally, she was sort of saying, well she was sort of more on Edward's side. Not on his side, but thinking that he was right and that he shouldn't be on a section. But as I say the next time she rang me, she said 'I didn't realise how ill your son was'. She said that she'd been to see him again and had spent time with him and that she understood now why I was so worried. Anyway she was away on leave, so there was another solicitor standing in, who'd not met Edward before and only had the notes. The social worker who was involved in his care couldn't be there, so someone else was standing in. The only person who was there who knew Edward and had actually met him before was Edward's consultant and he came back from holiday with his family to be there. He felt that strongly that Edward should be kept on section and wanted in fact to up the section to section 3 so that he could give him medication, because Edward wasn't complying at the time.

The review was at 10.00 am on the 29th and I arrived at about half past 9 with Nigel.. Sometime later, about fifteen minutes or so, a guy came in and then went off again. Then the CPN came in and asked us to come up and we collected Edward on the way. One odd thing I remember was that Edward had asked for his new shoes. The old shoes he had were falling to bits and he said to me 'I'm going to need to look smart for this court thing' – he rang me the morning before and said 'Have you got the shoes you bought me for Christmas?' and when I'd said 'yes', he'd asked me to bring them. So I took the shoes in, but in fact it all happened so quickly, that throughout the review Edward ended up with his shoes on that were falling into bits and I was holding a pair of white trainers. Anyway, we went in …and….I'd never….well I didn't know what to expect. I didn't know what it was like. We were sitting on one side and there were three people on the other side of the table. They introduced themselves and the chap who said he was the chairman introduced himself, he didn't have much to say really. The lady next to him didn't say a word, she just nodded when she was introduced. There was a doctor, an independent doctor who basically ran things and Edward of course, who for the first time for ages had complied with medication and kept falling asleep. He'd taken it the night before and they nurses had to wake him up for the review and he wasn't quite with it. Edward's consultant put up a very, very good case, he explained what Edward was like. How the nurses had reported to him the day before that he was laughing and talking to himself and throwing things at the television…and that….something else he'd done, I can't remember what it was, but the nurses were aware of it. His GP had written and said that he'd been to see him and that Edward was not the Edward he knew and that you know, he felt he was very ill. They got all the bits together and then we were asked to leave while they discussed it. The solicitor said to me 'Perhaps you'd like to go downstairs and have a coffee because these things take time' and Nigel had said

307

he'd go down to have a cigarette because he was still smoking at the time. Edward had decided that he wasn't going anywhere. I said to the solicitor, 'it's okay, I'll stay here with Ed'. That's when he changed his shoes and we threw the old ones in the bin. We weren't there very long - the solicitor was still there - when we were all called back again. We went back into the room and the doctor just said that they were lifting the sectioning. That they didn't think Edward should be sectioned. 'You can take him home', he said. He hadn't seen Edward before at all. He'd read his notes, he had 15 minutes to read his notes, I found that out afterwards. Nigel had not even finished his cigarette when we went back in there, that was how long they spent considering it. Just like that he said 'You can take him home'. I said 'I'm not taking him home. I don't think he's well enough. I think he needs to be in hospital. I can't cope with somebody like Edward at the moment. I wouldn't know how to handle it'. I said 'I really think he needs to be in hospital, so I'm not taking him home'. Actually I swore at them all, and I've never done that in public before. I went out really upset, and the CPN or somebody or other, I can't remember exactly took me downstairs for a cup of tea and we met Nigel coming back and I told him what had happened. He couldn't believe it.

It was then that the CPN told me that the doctor had only arrived 15 minutes before the hearing and hadn't really had time even to look at Edward's notes and didn't even have a chance to meet Edward. I was extremely upset. And because Edward wasn't sectioned he was allowed to go out and about. He obviously had to stay in hospital because he didn't have anywhere else to go, I'd refused to have him at home. It did cause....sort of....not a rift exactly, but it caused something between Edward and I. Like he didn't feel as though he had a home, I suppose. I think he felt I rejected him, even though I still went in to see him every day. He just felt that I didn't want him. I found that quite painful.

I wrote to the review board and complained. I also sent a letter to the doctor – I didn't know his name, but I sent it to the review board and I said that if anything ever happened to my son I would put the blame on him, because Edward had needed treatment and he wasn't getting it. I got a reply from the board – I never had a reply from the doctor and I'm not surprised – which basically said that mentally ill patients, or patients who are considered mentally ill, are allowed to hold these reviews and that was how it should be. That the decision should be upheld and they were sure it was run properly and everything else. Strangely enough though, when Edward put in for one the next year, the medical people at the hospital asked me to write to ask that they would ensure I had a correct...that I had one held correctly, with the correct proceedings. So they were aware it wasn't right and I know the nurses were quite upset and shocked by what had happened.

Edward ended up staying in hospital till March, when he suddenly decided he was going to discharge himself. His CPN found him a room in a bed and breakfast and rung up and said 'Joy, this is Edward's new address'. I rung up Richard and said that I thought we should go and see Edward. We went out there and it was the most horrific place. He had a dingy, dirty little room. A door hanging off the cupboard, the bedding on the bed was filthy and horrible. There was a dirty sink in the corner. There was as a fridge - the only thing that looked decent was the fridge - that was clean. There was a wardrobe but all the hanging things were broken and on the floor so you couldn't actually put anything in the wardrobe. Edward was just sitting on the bed staring. I think he'd probably been sitting there since his CPN had left him. He didn't seem to know what to do. So we went out together and brought him everything he needed. Bedding, towels, cooking utensils, food. Everything. We tried to set him up in a home. To make him feel comfortable and to have everything he needed.

Over the next lot of weeks, we – Emma and I mostly – went over there every day. Taking him to Social Services, finding a new GP and getting him into, or trying to find out where all the drop-in places were. He used to go to one or two of them for a bit. It was while I was doing this research and trying to find out all these things, that I found out about a Carer Support Worker and that was my breakthrough to everything. She was brilliant. She understood just how much fear I had for Edward and how vulnerable he was and she... she told me so many things that I didn't know and explained so many things I didn't understand. I saw her, you know, quite a few times and it was such a relief to talk to her and we – Nigel came with me at times as well – found out so many things. She was trying to see if she could get him into a place nearby which was sort of a halfway house, it had support and things. She was trying to see if there was a space there for him, trying to get that sorted out when Edward started to go downhill again. I mean he wasn't well when he was in the Bed and Breakfast. We all knew he wasn't well and that he should still have been in hospital. It was getting worse. A chap called Bob had the room next door, a nice old chap really. He was an alcoholic so he used to take Edward out drinking and then when Edward talked about cannabis, he said his son smoked cannabis and he took Edward round to his son's, that got Edward got back onto cannabis again. The delusions came back in full swing then and the fear started. He was different when we used to go round to take him out in the car. He'd have his collar pulled right up and he'd look out the door very scared and rush into the car quickly because he didn't want to be outside in the open.

That....that was one of the first signs really of Edward becoming ill; the fear. Of being watched and having to be careful.

At the time his brother had opened a shop in Cheltenham and we had, we were going to have a nice family trip– me, Emma, James and Edward - to look at the shop and then I was going to take them out to lunch and treat them. I was really looking forward to it spending time with all my children, all together. Then Edward said he wasn't going to come and so it was just going to be the three of us. At 9 o'clock in the morning, he rang up and said 'I want to come Mum' and I said, 'Well okay, we'll pick you up on the way through'. At quarter past nine he rang again and said 'Where are you? I'm still waiting'. I hadn't even left the house yet, I was still waiting for his brother *(laughs)*....So his concept of time and everything was way out.

Anyway, we got to Cheltenham. All the way travelling there, Edward was smiling and laughing to himself and kind of, not talking, but whispering now and then. We sort of ignored it going there. When we got to where the shop was, Edward refused to get out of the car so the other two and I went and had a look round the shop and then went back to the car. Then we went to a multi-storey car park and parked because it was near the shopping area and we knew there were some places to eat there. Again Edward wouldn't get out of the car and said that he was going to stay there. In the end we weren't happy about leaving him sitting there all on his own, I was a bit worried. I went off and bought some sandwiches and drinks and we just travelled back. On the way back, Edward was still laughing to himself and things and James said, 'What's the joke Ed? Come on share it. Let's all have a laugh.' Edward got quite annoyed and said 'It's none of your business. Why should I tell you anything? I don't have to tell you things. I can laugh privately if I want to.' So James said 'Ok, ok, fine. Course you can.' *(laughs)* We just left it at that.

We got him back home and dropped him off and I phoned his CPN and said to him, 'I'm really worried about Edward. There's something seriously wrong, I think he's really going downhill again'. He said that he'd call round and see him. He tried to but he couldn't, Edward wouldn't let him in. He had to speak to him through the door. In the end it ended up with the CPN and the consultant psychiatrist (who actually left the hospital to come down and talk to Ed) trying to tell Edward that he needed to be back in hospital. Edward still wouldn't accept it and they had to call the police and again he was taken back into hospital by the police. As soon as the police came, he did as they told him. He...he was always, well when it came to authority, he never went against it, he never argued with it. He just...well his attitude was 'if that's what I've got to, then that's what I've got to do' sort of thing. So he went back into hospital and they put him on Section 3 this time because he still wouldn't comply with medication. They started giving him injections and slowly, he started to improve.

It was amazing actually; Edward really started to come back. We went to a music event that was organised in a local park. That was one of his first outings. Emma and I went there with him and we spent well, most of the day there....um Edward found it hard at times. I think he found the crowd difficult and he used to have to sit down every so often, he'd go quite white and get a bit shaky. I think it was just sort of, a panicky feeling, because there were a lot of people and things. We kept close to him, Emma was on one side of him and I was on the other. He was waiting for Samantha Mumba who he thought was absolutely wonderful *(laughs)*. Emma and I were getting hungrier and hungrier and we kept offering Edward food. And Ed - well the other thing about Ed was that he never wanted to be a bother - he always felt that he didn't want to make a nuisance of himself, to be any trouble. So he kept saying 'no, no I'm alright, I'm alright'. In the end I said to Emma, 'it's no good, I'm going to have to go and get some chips, I'm really starving' and so Emma said, 'Oh yeah, I'll get something as well.' Then Edward pipes up 'Can I have something?' *(laughs)* So all the time that he was saying I'm alright, he wasn't, he actually wanted something to eat as well. He just didn't want to be a bother. That was Edward really. Anyway we all got some food and we saw Samantha Mumba, then took him back and it was a nice day out really.

At that time as well, he went out with the hospital for an outing. They went to a wildlife park and he brought me back a picture of a tiger and two cubs – I've got it framed in the other room – and it says something ...um, it says 'You can't beat a loving family.' So that...that always chokes me up when I see it, because...it ...it meant a lot....'um for Edward to pick that out and give it to me, I thought it was really lovely. I think it was his way of saying I understand you're there for me sort of thing... *(pauses)*

When he was out of hospital between the two episodes, he'd been to the local further education college because he'd wanted to start to do his A-levels again. He was desperate to still go on to Art College and do A-levels. He'd taken his Art and things into the college and he'd actually been accepted. In the September when he was due to start, he was still in hospital. None of the mental health team let the college know that Edward had problems. I made an appointment and went and spoke to the college and explained what was happening, what, well you know that Edward may not be able to do what he was hoping to do, and also that he had mental health problems and may need a bit more support, or different treatment. That sometimes he may appear a bit odd or something and I felt that they needed to know. I met the college nurse who was also a psychiatric nurse and he was very understanding, very good and he said he wanted to see Edward. We took Edward in and he explained that he felt three A levels was rather a lot to try and do in one go. That he might not be as strong as he thought he was, but Edward was insistent. So the nurse agreed but said that he should bear it in mind, that he could drop one or two if he felt it was all getting a bit much. He also showed him a room and said 'This room here is for you, whenever you want to time out, whenever you feel pressured or if anything's too much just come in here. I'm not going to bother you unless you want to talk to me, but you can come here and go to sleep or just come and sit down.' He gave him a quiet place away from everything, I mean he was really good. Also the nurses at the hospital, well they used to make him a packed lunch to take and they were really, they were so nice. They would keep his meal if he was back late and that sort of thing. They did everything they could to make him feel comfortable.

Of course he felt uncomfortable being in hospital and going to college. He would worry about what to say if someone asked him where he lived or if he wanted to bring someone back. It was getting difficult. So when we next had a mental health meeting, and it was decided that though he would remain on sectioning for the meantime, he would move into a room into a halfway house.

We worked out a system where Monday and Tuesday he would be at college, Wednesday I met him after work and we would go out for a meal; sometimes on our own, sometimes with the family. Sometimes we went to the cinema as well, to see a film as well as have a meal. But we did something every Wednesday evening. On a Thursday, Nigel used to collect him at lunchtime and take him to where he worked, which is just over the road from here, a residential home for old people. Edward used to help picking up leaves because autumn time was coming, he cleared up leaves and did a bit of gardening. He got to know quite a few of the elderly ladies over there, and they were always making him cups of tea or bringing him out lemonade and things, and he used to chat with them. He would do the same thing on Fridays. Nigel used to call up to him Friday mornings. Quite often he wouldn't want to get up and Nigel used to say, 'Yup come on up you get' and he would end up going. Saturday he'd spend the day here and then Sunday or Saturday evening sometimes he would go over and spend it with his dad. So it..., everything was really working, and was very structured.

I had a really good day out with him in Reading around this time. He needed some new clothes – he'd destroyed so many things and given so many away – for college and so we went shopping and we had a lovely day out. A really, really nice day. Quite exceptional because he was really happy and he was enjoying looking at clothes and enjoying buying them and trying them on and things. It was better than anything we'd done for ages. I saw a skirt in a window that I liked, and he said, 'Go on Mum, go and try it on' and he came with me while I tried it on and I bought it in the end. I've still got it, the skirt, upstairs.

Then in October, Nigel and I were due to go away on holiday and because he'd moved and his regular CPN had gone on long term sick, it was decided that he needed to change to a different mental health team. Basically his regular mental health team broke down and Daryl, who was the warden of the house he was staying, was more or less handed Edward to sort of, take care of until there was a proper support team in place. It wasn't Daryl's responsibility really and though he did as best he could, he was in an awkward position. He worked for housing support group and had 7 other people that he looked after. He had the running of the house to take care of. Organising taking them out and doing things and stuff so it didn't work very well...

Edward started dropping out of odd classes at college again. For his art class he was put into a class of 16 year old girls, there were no other males in there, which

Edward found quite alarming. I think even somebody who wasn't mentally ill, any young man would have found that alarming. The college probably thought it was a gentle thing to do but I think he would have been a lot happier if he'd been put in with a load of lads that talked the same music and things than with all these girls *(laughs)*. But that's where he ended up. The other two classes: one was media studies and I can't remember what the other subject was that he was doing but slowly he'd dropped out of them because he couldn't handle them.

The first day he started the art class, when he joined the girls in the art class, he came back and he borrowed Nigel's razor and he shaved his head. He went back to when he was about fifteen, he'd had his head shaved then. He wanted it to be like that again. Then on the Monday because he was here for the week, I'd given him some money for his lunch. He didn't want a packed lunch, he said he wanted to buy it and so I'd given him some money. He came back home that day really, really upset and depressed because he'd had his ear pierced and he wished he hadn't done it, and he wished he hadn't shaved his hair off. I felt ever so sorry for him because I think he didn't get the reaction he wanted. He'd done this when he'd gone to college before you see when he was one of the boys. He wanted everything to be like that again and it didn't actually work this time.

One of the other things I'd done, was that I'd also found Kirsty's phone number and I rang her and I told her about Edward and about how ill he was. She rang him and she spoke to him a few times on the phone. She actually said to me, she said, 'I was really, really fond of Edward', I said 'Yes I thought you were'. She that she hadn't been able to cope with his drinking, he had been drinking so heavily in London, she said she just hadn't been able to cope with it. That he'd been very difficult and when he'd been drinking she just couldn't reason with him. I think it was more than just the alcohol that she was trying to deal with. Anyway they had arranged to meet in Reading and I think she travelled from Tunbridge Wells to Reading and Edward didn't go. He wouldn't go, he stood her up. They never actually got back together again and I felt quite sad about that because I think they…well she probably wouldn't have been a girlfriend, but she would have been a good friend. Someone who would have been there for him and would have listened to him. That was something I was quite sad about, that it didn't work out.

Anyway, Nigel and I went away to Malta for a couple of weeks and when we came back Edward was different. He was very down again. All his motivation had gone. He didn't want to come and work with Nigel anymore. He didn't want to come and meet me on Wednesdays for dinner, though Emma had seen him while we were away and taken him out a few times. We did try. We even took him to see 'Bridget Jone's Diary' and *(laughs)* he absolutely hated it. He sat there really, really cross. So that was a mistake...For his birthday in November, he wanted another pair of trainers and the trip to Reading that day was, well it was an evening after work and was completely different to the one trip I'd done with him before. I've never rushed through shoes in shops so quickly. He knew what he was looking for but he was so ill that he didn't want to be out, he didn't want to be in the open. He just shot into the shops, looked along the shelves very quickly and marched out. I was running to keep up with him. I mean he was six foot and with him walking fast, it was quite hard for me to keep up with my little tubby legs *(laughs)*. Eventually we found the right ones, bought them and went straight back to the car. I said 'Shall we have a meal or something? Or go for a drink?' But he was adamant he wanted to go straight back home. Emma was with us and she was shocked. People were looking, you know, in the shops, not because he looked peculiar or anything, but because he was rushing so much. They were probably thinking 'Well if you're buying shoes, what's the rush?' *(laughs)*.

I was beginning to get quite alarmed again at that point. I spoke to Daryl, the warden at the halfway house and said that I was really worried about him. He said that he wasn't sure if Edward was taking his meds. He thought that he was probably taking enough to keep him on an even keel but not taking them properly. He wasn't really sure what to do, that he could just see him going downhill. He said 'It's a shame he can't have those injections again because they were really working'. Apparently he was spending more and more time in his room. He didn't want to go bowling with them or do any of the things, the activities that they were sorting out. The staff used to go in and play board games and things with them and stuff. They had a billiards table there and things. Edward used to enjoy playing that but he didn't want to do that anymore. He wouldn't stay down with them to watch television or anything. He was just up in his room the whole time.

At this time, I used to go and visit and there would be quite a strong smell of cannabis in the house. Daryl was aware of it. He said that he knew one of the boys was getting it, and that he knew which one it was. Unfortunately he wasn't allowed to go into their rooms. If they were smoking in the communal area he could have stopped them. Their room is their place he said and that he couldn't intervene in whatever they were doing in there. He could talk to them about it and things but that's as far as it could go. But it was…I knew the lad, I can't remember his name but I knew the lad that was doing it. I'd go there sometimes and Edward would be in this room and he wouldn't want to see me. Anyway it was obviously not doing him any good. I can remember phoning a social worker, not his assigned social worker, because he still didn't have a mental health team. She wasn't able to look after Edward as such because her books were full, but she used to, if I had a problem, she'd come out and see him and she'd talk to Edward and she'd talk to me. She came out to see him because I was worried. Eventually she arranged just before Christmas, a mental health review, not a review exactly, but a sort of carer's meeting. We all went, Daryl, Edward, myself, Nigel and his consultant. We talked it all over again Nobody could understand why the new mental team was taking so long and the social worker agreed to write to them again to see if they could get some sort of action. The consultant talked to Edward about having injections again and said 'They worked for you last time Edward and you were really good and well, will you have them again?' At that time Edward kind of agreed, and said 'yes'. When the social worker picked him up on the Monday to take him to his GP and when they got there the GP didn't have the right sort of stuff in, so he didn't get the injection. By the time the new appointment was made and the stuff had arrived, Edward wouldn't move, he refused to have it. That was another mess up, another missed opportunity. I wished the consultant had been able to give it to him there and then at the meeting. The injection lasts for a few weeks you see, and it would have started to work and then they could have given him another one.

By Christmas he was really quite poorly. He was hearing voices and he kept headphones on all the time, playing music, trying to block out the voices. He came here for Christmas. He was....he was quite sweet, but he couldn't sleep. As I said, he had these headphones on all the time and he wasn't sleeping, he was fidgeting all night. Nigel and I didn't get any sleep Christmas Eve and on Christmas Day we were pretty tired. On Christmas night I said to Edward 'Do you mind if we take you home and pick you up tomorrow morning?' I said, 'I know you're not sleeping and it's stopping us sleeping and Nigel and I don't feel very well because we've not had any sleep'. He understood and agreed and we took him over to his place. At that time there was another boy, Chris, who Edward was very friendly with; who was also smoking cannabis and not sleeping. The rest of the people in the place where they were living were complaining because these two weren't sleeping and it was keeping them awake. Anyway the whole of that week, between Christmas and New Year, we were ferrying Edward backwards and forwards.

Then just after New Year he phoned up his dad and said 'Can you take me to Marlow?' and Richard said 'Why?'. Edward said 'Because my girlfriend's very ill, she's been raped and she's seriously ill in hospital'. Richard rang me and I said 'Well he hasn't got a girlfriend and I don't even know if there's a hospital in Marlow'. He said that Edward had said that his girlfriend was intensive care. Richard didn't really know what to do so I said to ring him and tell him you're not taking him tonight, because he wouldn't be allowed in as he's not family. To sort of see what he said the next day. By the next morning, things weren't so bad. He'd told his Dad that this girl was going to be in intensive care for at least six months, she was so seriously ill, then when I saw him later that day and I said 'Oh, how's this girlfriend then?' He said 'Oh, she's alright, she's coming out of hospital tomorrow' (laughs). So we knew then, that whatever was going on, well it was....I knew it was all in his head anyway.

I then wrote a letter to the new mental health people. I just addressed it to the Mental Health Team. I explained to them what had happened to Edward, where he'd become ill, what had happened then and that now he was in complete limbo. He wasn't getting any proper mental health support and I didn't know what to do to help him. I was doing as much as I could. I felt we both needed more support with what was happening. I asked them exactly what was I supposed to do? That the old mental health team had been writing to them and nothing happened. Did they want me to take Edward and take him to back to Stevenage and just drop him there (because that's where he became ill) before they dealt with it? Or was he going to be taken care of where he'd been born and bred? That was …. I suppose sometime in February because I got a letter very soon after inviting me to a carer's meeting on the 28th February. That was the first time I met his new consultant and the people who were going to be Edward's mental health team. The social worker who'd been helping us most recently was there, Daryl was there, his old consultant couldn't make it unfortunately but they had all his notes anyway. His new consultant saw us and then he saw Edward. He asked Edward to wait outside and he said to us 'I had a few words with Edward earlier, before you arrived. I don't think he's very well and I don't think him sitting in on this meeting would do him any good. So I've asked him to wait outside'. While he was talking to us about Edward, Edward was listening outside the door and opened the door and came in saying: 'I'm not going back into hospital'. The consultant had been saying that he thought Edward needed to be brought back into hospital to stabilise his medication. He said 'So that's my plan'. He'd just come down from Scotland, he was new there and apparently the rules in Scotland are different to what they are down here. The social worker and Edward's new CPN turned round and said 'You can't do that'. When he asked why and they said that he wasn't yet a danger to himself or to other people and so he couldn't be made to go into hospital. He needed a proper assessment and things. This was quoted at me so many times, this thing about being a danger to yourself and a danger to someone else, that one of my arguments is that by that time it's surely that's too late. You've either harmed yourself or you've harmed someone else before it's decided that something needs to be done. They were saying 'On no, no, no, he has to be assessed before he's admitted' and all this sort of thing and Edward opened the door and just said 'I'm not going into hospital'. The consultant tried to convince him to go in, that it would probably only be for two weeks, then he could go back home. Maybe not even that, he said but he (the consultant) needed to get to know him a bit more and work on his medication. Edward said 'There's nothing wrong with me, I'm perfectly alright. Actually I'm fine. I don't know what's wrong with the rest of you, but I'm ok and I'm not coming in'. And he walked out. His consultant just sort of looked at all of us and said 'We've got to wait for him to crash have we?' and they all said yes.

I tried to talk to his new CPN, but she was, well, she was very standoffish, not very friendly and very dismissive. She didn't want to discuss Edward with me and she never, ever, during the time from February, well it was only till March but she never asked me about Edward's history. What sort of person he was, never...nothing... I think perhaps she wasn't as confident as she seemed. I mean maybe she was new in the job, I don't know. I know some professionals don't like parents or friends involved, which I find really weird because they're the people that actually know the people who are sick....but she....she was very standoffish. Almost gave me the feeling that she thought she was superior to me. His consultant was much more down to earth.

We struggled on in March. Emma had a birthday and we asked Edward if he wanted to join us because we were going to a Thai restaurant and he didn't. It was my mum's 80th birthday the week before he died and that weekend we had a party in Essex where she lived. We asked Edward and he didn't want to come to that. He was polite but standoffish at the time. Not wanting to know anybody, not wanting to be involved. He wasn't even involved with any of the people in the house. Chris, his friend in the house, had by then been taken into hospital. I think without Chris he felt a bit lost anyway, although he did know the others. Daryl and Hilda, who were the staff in the house, said that he was coming out of his room while they were there but not staying out and going back quite quickly. The others were saying they weren't seeing him at all. I could never get him on the phone. Quite often I would ring and he wouldn't come to the phone. I felt quite sorry for one of the older guys in particular who always seemed to answer the phone. He was getting cross - I could hear it in his voice - and I used to apologise. I felt I needed to try each day in case one day he would come and talk. When I used to go round there, whoever opened the front door, well they'd go up and knock on his door and he wouldn't come out. Sometimes I'd go in the house and knock on his door and talk to him through the door and sometimes he wouldn't answer me properly. So it was just a... a battle.

Anyway I managed to talk to him on the Thursday, Maundy Thursday, and said 'The family are coming round on Easter Sunday, are you coming over to stay for Easter? Are you going to join us for a family meal?' He said no, that he was going to stay at his house. After I put the phone down, because he sounded so sort of sharp, like he did when he'd been at Simon and Sue's, I phoned the hospital and asked to talk to his consultant. I didn't get hold of him but I did end up talking to someone who worked in the house, Hilda, a support worker. She sort of said that he seemed ok, that she'd seen him and that he'd been quite sharp but very polite, that he was spending most of his time in his room. I appreciated her ringing but at the end of the day she was a support worker, her training was probably not much more than mine. I wanted to talk to somebody more professional. I couldn't get hold of his CPN although I had spoken to her about two weeks before. She'd called into see him for about 5 minutes, so Daryl said because he used to have to sit in on their meetings. Edward was by then talking in this - when you did manage to talk to him that is– in an American, a

329

black American rap type voice. I asked her if he'd been talking in that weird voice and she said yes. I said that I thought that he thought he was a rapper. She said 'Oh, I don't think so, they're all into rap music at his age'. I said 'Yes but I think it's more than that. I think Edward actually thinks he is a rapper' and she said 'No, no, he may be a little delusional but he's alright. It's nothing to worry about.' She made me feel, I don't know, like I didn't know what I was talking about.

I'd also had another conversation with Daryl about Edward's medication. At one point he tried to go into his room to see if he was taking it, he wasn't allowed to really but he phoned the housing agency, his employer, and they gave him permission as long as he spoke to me about it first. I said that it was fine with me. So when Edward had gone out, Daryl had gone into the room and he hadn't been in there for more than two minutes when Edward came back again and caught him in the room. When Edward asked what he was doing there, Daryl told him the truth, that he was checking to see whether he was taking his meds. Edward said 'Well I am' and that was that. Unfortunately that incident destroyed some of the trust between the two of them. But when Edward died we found a pile of repeat prescriptions in his drawer.

Anyway on Easter Saturday, Edward suddenly rung up at about half past five and said 'Mum, can I come home? Can I come and stay for Easter?' and I said 'Of course. You know that's what we want'. We went and collected him. He was…he was very quiet, quite calm and different. I knew he wasn't well…there…because he wasn't actually himself, but I couldn't put my finger on what was different about him. He was much friendlier that he had been but there was something different and I just didn't know what it was. We had his favourite meal, which was steak and chips and then we started to watch a video. At one point he got up and he went outside, I thought he'd gone out for a cigarette. He was gone for so long though that I went outside and he was sat at the desk writing and when I came in he screwed the bit of paper up and put it in his pocket. Nigel had gone up to bed when Edward came back in and said he was going upstairs because he'd wanted to listen to some rap music on the radio. He came down about half an hour later and said the music wasn't on, that all he could find was classical music. We eventually figured out it was because the Queen Mother had died and they'd cancelled his rap programme. We sat for a while and we chatted about rap music and about him wanting to be a rapper and how he could…we tried to work out how he could get himself known and things and talked about perhaps getting some money together and him doing a demo and things….Then he got up to go to bed and he said 'I love you mum'. I said 'I love you Ed', and he went upstairs and I tidied up in here. I went upstairs, heard him go back downstairs and say that he was going down to take his medication. I fell asleep and about half past two in the morning there was a bang on my door and he flung the door open and he stood there, in his jeans, he didn't have a top on and his chest was covered in blood and he had a cut right across his throat, one of skin bit hanging down. I just woke up with a start and he said 'Mum, I've tried to kill myself. I've cut my throat'.

I really, honestly can't explain how I felt. I was shaking and panicking. I just burst downstairs because we didn't have a phone upstairs, and phoned the psychiatric hospital. I couldn't think. I tried to tell them what he'd done because obviously he was one of their patients. I wasn't thinking straight. They said to phone the surgery. I said 'it's half past two on Easter Sunday morning, there's nobody in the surgery. Then Nigel yelled downstairs 'Phone the fucking ambulance, phone for a fucking ambulance'. And I did.

They were very good, the people on the other end of the line. I explained what he'd done and they told me how to treat him and to get Nigel outside to wait for the ambulance, so that the paramedics would be able to find the house. I knelt with Edward, holding one of his hands and talking to him and he gave me this suicide note. It was what he'd been writing at the desk earlier. He was talking a lot, telling me that he thought three men were coming. That he'd been having an affair with another rapper's wife and that all the rappers had found out and they'd employed these three men from London. They were coming down to torture him in the most horrific way they could and they were going to slowly kill him. The voices were telling him that he needed to kill himself before these men got him. He kept saying 'Mum, I'm really, really scared, I don't want to die'. I kept saying 'Edward, I don't want you to die, you're ill, you need help'. When he said he was going to get his medication he'd gone to the kitchen and taken a knife because he thought he'd heard these men outside the house and that they were going to come and get him. The ambulance people – the paramedics – patched him up and said that he needed stitching. They didn't allow him to be alone, they didn't even allow him to go in the garden to smoke a cigarette. I went in the ambulance with him to the A and E and Nigel stayed here and phoned Richard and Emma and that, to let them know what had happened.

At the hospital he was still quite agitated and in fact the doctor came in and said to him 'You're very agitated Edward, what's wrong?'. Edward told him about what he thought was happening and he said 'Well not to worry, nobody's going to come in here'. Edward was panicking and said 'Well what if they do, what if they come in?' and he said

'Nobody's allowed in without giving their names and saying who they want to see and we will come and ask you when they come, to see if you want to see them. If you don't, they're not allowed to.' That sort of calmed Edward a little bit. He had 3 or 4 internal stitches and a lot of stitches across the outside and then they put steri-stitches on because it was in such a sort of, awkward place. The doctor was quite sweet and he said to Edward 'I've stitched you in such a way that there won't be a scar. I've used dissolving stitches and it will just look like you've got a crease in your neck. He said that nobody would need ever know what Edward had done which I thought was really, you know, a nice thing to do.

All the time Edward was in the ward there he was never ever left on his own. All the time he was there, they never left him. There was always a nurse there if I needed to go off somewhere or else they knew I was with him. He was assessed by the duty psychiatrist quite quickly. She was very good, she was with Ed for about an hour and we sat in on it. Richard was with us by then and Emma. She sort of said to him 'Edward, what if I told you that no men, no people are coming from London. That there's nothing like that ever going to happen and nobody's going to harm you' ,and he said

'I know that's what you believe, I know that's what mum believes and my sister and my dad. But to me it's real. To me it's going to happen and I'm really, really scared'.

And she said, 'Yes, I know you are and you need to be in hospital'.

He said 'Yes, I know. I know I'm mentally ill'.

She said 'Well, we're going to see if we can sort it out. I'll try to contact the psychiatric hospital and see when we can get you a bed. She went off and we had to wait for ages. Not because of her, she'd phoned the hospital and faxed over all Edward's details but the doctor she spoke had said 'I'll get back to you in ten minutes' and it had been over an hour and ten minutes, when she had to ring again. Again he said I'll get back to you in ten minutes time and it was then, well nearly another hour before he actually got back to us and they accepted him.

We started to take him over to the hospital. On the way he wanted a sandwich and a drink, but as it was Easter Sunday and everywhere was shut. I said that he'd be better off waiting till we got to the hospital because it was getting on for teatime. When we got there we were given directions through…oh…through corridors, upstairs, down lifts…all sorts of places till we got to this ward. It was a chaotic place, we didn't know who was a nurse, who was a doctor, who were the patients, people were just milling around. It was very untidy, we couldn't see a nurses' station or a sign up that said 'New patients please report here', or anything like that. Eventually I spoke to this guy who was standing around with a clipboard and he didn't answer me, he just directed us over to a room and we followed him. There was a nurse in there and she directed us into another room and said she'd let the doctor know. We sat in there and waited and she kept putting her head round the door and apologising for us having to wait so long. Eventually the doctor arrived and the guy with the clipboard came in. He still wasn't introduced, but by then we'd presumed he was a nurse. The doctor introduced himself and he sat opposite me, next to Edward, and I explained what had happened; I told him about the neck injury and I also tried to fill him in on Edward's medical details.

And he said 'Oh well yes don't worry, I've got the notes'. I went to give him the suicide note and he said 'Oh, that's the joined up, the big joined up writing letter is it?'

So I said 'Yes' and he said 'Oh, I've had a faxed copy of that'. So I put that back in my bag. Then he looked at Edward and he said

'If you had a gun, would you use it?'

Edward just looked at him and said 'Why would I want a gun? Where would I get a gun from?'

The doctor didn't answer and said 'So he did this yesterday morning did he?'

We said 'No, he did it this morning'.

336

'Oh right so you guys have had no sleep?'

We said 'no' and he turned round to Edward and said

'Don't you think they've suffered enough?'

Edward didn't answer and he said

'I think we ought to let them go home now, don't you? I think they can go home'.

I said 'I'd rather stay until Edward's settled in thank you'.

He said again to Edward

'You don't need them here now. They can go home can't they? I think they should go home. They've been through enough. They've suffered enough'.

I could see Edward getting quite stressed and I said 'Look, if we've got to go home, we'll go'. I said

'Edward, I'll be in first thing to see you tomorrow morning' and

Edward said 'ok'.

The doctor said

'You don't want your mum here in the morning. She can have the day off. Go on, you can give your mum a day off can't you? She doesn't need to come tomorrow'.

Edward said 'No, I want to see my mum',

and I said 'I'll be here, don't worry. I'll come in the morning and see you'. His dad said he'd be there as well and Emma said the same. So we were all agreed that we were going to come and see him.

Then the doctor said 'Right, ok, there's just one tiny thing. We may have to move you and send you to another hospital'.

Edward became really alarmed at this point then and said 'What do you mean, what do you mean?'.

The doctor said 'Oh, well, it's not necessary. It may not happen. I just said it's one tiny little thing, but it may not happen. I'm not saying it's going to, you'll probably stay here. It was just a little warning, just in case'. Edward still looked panicky and the doctor said 'But don't worry, I'm sure it won't happen. We'll sort you out here.'

Then he got up and he walked out and the guy with the clipboard walked out and we all just sat there and looked at each other and said 'What now?' Edward was so agitated and worked up by what had happened that he got up and walked outside, so we followed him out. The guy with the clipboard was stood outside and I said

'What are we supposed to do now? Have we got to go or can we stay?'

And he said 'No, you should go'.

I said to Edward - I hugged him – and I said I loved him and not to worry that we would be there first thing in the morning. Then his dad said goodbye and Emma said goodbye. We got to the door and I looked back and he was standing there. He was near to tears and he had this bag over his back. He looked so forlorn. My gut instinct was to say 'Come on Ed, come home'. I didn't because logic said that he was in the place that he needed to be. That they'd be able to give him medication and be able to help him and I wasn't able to do that. So we left and we went got home. It was about half past five and Nigel said "Come on, we need a drink" and we went to the pub for a drink. When I got back there was a message on the phone from Richard asking me to ring him. When I did and he said that he'd phoned the hospital at six o'clock to see if Edward had settled in and they couldn't find him, that he was missing. He said that James was out looking for him and that he (Richard) had already been out searching but was about to go out again. He told me to stay where I was just in case Edward tried to make his way here. He said that the hospital had been round to his flat but that he wasn't there. That the police were out and that they were talking about getting helicopters. He promised to let me know as soon as he heard anything.

I was just on edge, terrified. I didn't know what to do. I was just waiting, waiting. Just after nine, Richard rang again. He said that he was at the psychiatric hospital and that the police had just come in. There'd been someone who'd fallen from the multi-storey car park in Reading station. He said that they didn't know it was Edward but that there was a possibility. The description sounded like it might be him. He'd been taken to a hospital in Reading. I just...I... I think I just went "Oh no'. I told Nigel what had happened and rang my daughter. I'd asked Richard to pick us up because we'd been out drinking, and we all went and collected Emma. She followed us in her car because she didn't know the way to the hospital.

When we got there, James and Julia (James's girlfriend) who'd been out Reading way looking for Edward were already there. They were both crying. James just said:

It's Ed Mum...they've just asked if he had stitches to his neck. They've just taken him for a scan".

They were both in tears At that time I was absolutely stunned; I didn't know what to expect, I didn't know what had happened. I didn't know how far he'd fallen or anything. I mean, I didn't know if it was from the top that he fell, what floor it was. Opposite me there was a poster that said '1 in 8 people suffer from mental illness' and it gave a list of symptoms. It said 'If you're a family or a friend, don't leave it too late to get help'. I just ripped this poster off the wall and I put it in my handbag, and in fact a couple of days later, in a great big red felt tip, I put 'We were there for him. Where were you?' and I sent it to the psychiatric hospital *(pauses)*...

After Edward had his scan a doctor came in and said "I have to tell you that your son is 95% close to death and that…that he's injured from the top of his head to the tip of his toes". 'He needs operations but we've got him stable at the moment, if you'd like to come through and see him…but I must warn you that he is… very badly injured. He's fallen on his face and the injuries are horrific. Please prepare yourself". (*crying*).

And I thought I had. I thought I'd seen enough casualties or things on television to expect something, something awful. But it was worse….the worst thing I've ever, ever seen in my life. It's something that I'll never, ever forget. I find it difficult to remember Edward – I have pictures and photographs everywhere, even at work – because of this image I have of him, this thing that flashes into my head all the time is how he was in the hospital. He was so huge and swollen, his nose wasn't in the right place. There was blood coming out of his ears, his eyes, his nose, his mouth…I…his skin colour was just….all bruising, just…it was…it was horrible. I never, ever knew a head, a face could swell that much. All his features were huge. The reason I knew it was Edward was because he got bitten by a dog when he was seven and the scar was still on his shoulder…and I saw that. It convinced me then and I knew it was Edward. All I could do was go 'Oh Edward, Edward' and I kept saying his name over and over again (*crying*).

When I got outside, Nigel came up and I just said "We've lost him. He's not going to survive this. I've lost him".

He cuddled me and then James and Julia went in and saw him and they came out really upset and in tears and we were all cuddling. Then Emma and Nigel went in and saw him and they were in tears when they came out. We were escorted up to a family room to wait while Edward went into the operating theatre. They were the people that were looking for the internal injuries and the doctor came out halfway through and explained that they were having trouble stopping him bleeding and that blood was seeping out of his...um they said they had him on a blood pressure machine to try and keep his blood pressure up. That they were doing all they could and that when they'd finished, the ...orthopaedic surgeons were going in to set his bones. He went back in and when he came out he said again that they'd done the best they could. They'd packed his liver and his stomach had been ruptured so they'd done things to his stomach and things. They ...he said he'd had 40 pints of blood so far, 'um....anyway, the orthopaedic people went in. They came out and you almost felt uplifted for a while until we really thought about who they were. You see they came out and they said 'Well, it's all gone very well, everything's ok', and of course it was, they were just setting bones. But er, for that...brief 5 or 10 minutes we were thinking "Oh good, things are getting better", and then we thought well no, they're just talking about his bones ...

After the orthopaedic people went in, the plastic surgeons went in and did what they could for him. They came back and they sort of said, you know, that they'd done as much as possible because he was swollen up, that he would need more surgery once the swelling had gone down.

After that I went home briefly to have a wash and change my clothes, because I'd been in them for nearly 24 hours. I had to take some things back to the hospital because I thought... I didn't know how long I was going to be there. Nigel stayed here and Emma took me back to the hospital. Nigel phoned my mum and various other members of the family to let them know what had happened. When I got back to the hospital I went straight in to see Edward. There was a group of people around him and they were all discussing him. The doctor came to me and he said that they were going to take him for another scan and he said, 'I must warn you, tell you that the trauma to Edward's body is horrific. If he survives this trauma, you know, it will be amazing". He said that there were so many injuries to him and although we should see how the scan went, not to, not to get our hopes up. I mean they were... they were very honest right from the beginning. They never gave us any false hopes, they were upfront the whole time and we knew what a risk it was. Anyway, Edward went off for another scan and a little while later a nurse asked if we could come and wait in a waiting room, in intensive care. There was a scan of a head on the wall and it was all lit up. I knew it was Edward and I said to Richard 'This is not going to be good news" but he, ever the optimist, said

"No, no it might not be Edward, it might be ok, it might be ok.".

But I think I knew right from the beginning when I first saw him, how bad it was. The doctor came in and he found it very difficult to tell us, he was very upset. He explained to us about the scan and how there was swelling at the top of Edward's head. That his brain had what they called 'coned', which was that it had seeped down into the neck, meaning that they hadn't been able to drill a hole to take away the pressure. He said that if he did survive all the trauma to his body, he would be so badly brain damaged that he would be in a vegetable state. So we had to make the decision… about what we wanted to do because he was being kept alive by machines.

It was very, very hard. Richard kept on and on at the doctor. That surely he must be able to do something, surely there was hope. Couldn't we leave it a bit and see? The doctor just kept saying no. As I say he was upset too. He said that they hated giving up on someone so young. The nurses were upset as well.

Eventually we all agreed that the best thing to do for Edward was to turn the machines off. We went in and we sat with him and we washed him and we held him and we talked to him the whole time. The nurse said that she felt that unconscious people can hear. She said that one of the last things to go is the hearing; and to just keep talking to him, which is what we did, telling him how much he was loved and how much we needed him.

Halfway through this a nurse put her head round the door and she said 'There's a phone call from the psychiatric hospital, they're asking how Edward is.' She said "I can't tell them because it's confidential, but if any of you would like to talk to her".

I was wound up and I said "I will". I went out and introduced myself and a woman said "We're just wondering how Edward is?" and I said "Well actually he's dying".

She said "Oh, I'm so sorry" and I replied that she should be. That he shouldn't be in here, that he should be there with them. Why wasn't he there with them?

She said "Well, we inadvertently lost him."

I said "What do you mean you inadvertently lost him?". I said "You should have been taking care of him." In the end I had to put the phone down because I couldn't talk to her anymore. I just said "I'm going back to my son, I can't listen to you" and I left.

I went back and sat with him. At some point Emma went out and rang Nigel to let him know what was happening and he joined us. We stayed with Edward until he died. He died at 3.24 pm that afternoon.

Then we had to go down to some stupid little room and talk to a nurse to about how we had to go and identify his body the next day with a coroner. They were talking about things going on with inquests and courts...and death certificates. I hadn't even taken in yet that Edward had died and you know, I know that's what they have to do...but it just...I wasn't ready for it. I wasn't ready for all of that. After we left there, we went and brought some flowers and we went to where Edward fell. He'd fallen, or rather jumped from the top of the car park. He fell about 40 feet. The police found a sandwich and an orange juice and his cigarettes at the top. We discovered afterwards that he'd bought a return ticket to Reading. We reckon what actually happened was that he didn't get anything to eat at the hospital, he'd actually asked to leave at one point and they'd said no. I think that was the time - because he'd gone in there voluntarily – that was the time he should have been sectioned, even if it was by nurses for 36 hours. But they didn't section him and he walked out. Anyway I think his original intention was to go to Reading, buy himself a sandwich and a drink and come back again. Somewhere along that line I think the voices started again, he felt this

346

fear again and he decided to go up and jump. He didn't eat the sandwich, he'd drunk some of the orange juice.

I left a message on the phone to his CPN reminding her about the conversation we had about Edward's delusions about rappers, when I said it wasn't just right. I left a message saying what had happened and I said "You may be the professionals, you may have read the books, you may have taken the exams, but you didn't know him and you never ever got to know him, and maybe you should listen to people who know the people who are ill."

One of my biggest fears, one of the things that upsets me more than anything - quite often I wake up in the night thinking about it and I get tearful - is that because when he cut his throat, he changed his mind and realised he wanted to live and he came to me for help... Well my biggest, biggest thing that I find hardest to cope with is the fact that he may have jumped off of that building and as he was falling, realised he didn't want to do it and that there was no going back. The fact that he broke both his elbows means he put his hands down to try and break his fall.

The other horrible thing that I think about sometimes as well is the fact that he was conscious when he went into hospital. He was trying to talk but they couldn't understand him (crying). That upsets me because I wasn't there, I wasn't there to talk to him, to tell him I was there, to tell him it was ok, that I loved him. I did talk to a nurse afterwards, a bereavement nurse I went to see. I could have gone to see her more but I couldn't cope with going back to the hospital at that time. She said, she said she that she went and checked Edward's records and she said that full consciousness was ranked at 15 and unconsciousness was ranked at 8 and Edward was reckoned to be about 12. So she said he wasn't ever fully conscious and he probably wasn't aware of his environment, which did comfort me to a point. But...I don't know whether she said that to make me feel better. She did say that they, they were all very shocked at the condition that he was in, what they'd seen. She was very good actually, she said she remembered Edward coming in and that she'd spoken to other nurses and they sedated him as quickly as they could. One of the first things they did was to sedate him...so he didn't suffer that much. But he must have suffered if he was conscious from the time they found him till the time he got to hospital, because obviously the paramedics couldn't give him anything...It's horrible. Horrible to think about.

There's a lot of things that went wrong. When my friend across the road heard what had happened – she used to be a psychiatric nurse – she said 'Ask for the, the sheet thing. The... the...observation sheet. Tell them you want a copy of the observation sheet'.

I rang them up, the day after it had happened, and I said "Can you let me have a copy of the observation sheet?". They said that they couldn't find his notes, that they didn't know where they were. They couldn't find them for two weeks or so they say. Eventually I did get an observation sheet and I showed it to my neighbour; it had:

'Edward - 5 o'clock - lying on his bed.'

(Well actually we didn't leave till 5 o'clock. He didn't have a bed then.)

'Quarter past 5 – asleep',

'Half past 5 - in the toilet,'

'Quarter to 6 - in the smoking room',

'Six o'clock – missing'.

So either he was very agitated and nobody saw anything because he was moving around an awful lot and nobody actually did anything about it, or they were making it up. From 6 o'clock every 15 minutes till...well for a whole day, they put 'missing', 'missing', 'missing', until he was actually found at nine o'clock. My neighbour said they wouldn't have done that, they wouldn't have every 15 minutes just gone and had a search round because they knew he wasn't there and they would have been out looking. She said usually if somebody goes AWOL they put 'missing' or 'AWOL' and then when they're found, they put the time in and details of where they're found. So all that seemed to be wrong.

At the inquest, the doctor who had admitted Edward was extremely arrogant. Very argumentative and quite sort of cocky, which was the feeling I had about him when I met him on that day. Edward's usual consultant actually went against him when he was questioned. He was asked if he thought Edward was on the wrong watch and he said 'yes', he should have been put on a much higher watch than 15 minutes. He was asked if he thought Edward's was a preventable death and he said that yes, he did think it was preventable. The coroner, in the end said that it was 'death by suicide while unbalanced of the mind, aggravated by lack of care.'

My solicitor told me that 'lack of care' is recognised by law. That it comes under negligence. So the lawyer's interpretation of it is 'death by suicide, while unbalanced of the mind, aggravated by negligence.' But that doctor, well he almost cheered when he heard the verdict. I don't know why, but they were all quite pleased because I think they were expecting negligence or they were expecting someone to be blamed for it and the coroner didn't go for that. He just...he went...I mean I don't even know if that's what coroners do. He actually said right at the beginning, "We're not here to find out the blame, we're here to find out what happened". So it was a long inquest. It started at 2 o'clock and we didn't actually leave until 7. We were all exhausted. Yes, it was a very long inquest.

His funeral was lovely, if you can say that. It was one of the hardest things I've ever had to do, to organise my own child's funeral, but it was the last, probably one of the last things I could do for Edward. Well this as well, I'm doing this interview for Edward. You want to do your last acts for your child. In his suicide note, he had said wanted to be cremated. I couldn't go and see him while he was in the Chapel Of Rest, I just couldn't go. In fact, I couldn't...go into the room when...to identify his body the day after he died. I couldn't, I just saw him from the door. I knew it was Edward. But Richard went, Richard went everyday while he was in the chapel of Rst.

Anyway the coffin... the coffin was brought into the village church, the village where we used to live, where Edward had lived. That was horrific, it was really...'um horrible. We had a few prayers there and then we travelled to the crematorium where we met my mum and my brother and Edward's cousins and other members of the family. My sister and things. After that we travelled back to the village where we had a memorial service. Well it wasn't a memorial service, it was more a celebration of his life. I wanted to do that. People kept saying 'Oh, don't do it on the same day', but I wanted it all done together. I was, I was amazed when I walked into the church because it was absolutely full. I mean really full. I mean there were over 100 people who came down to the reception and not all of the people in the church did. In fact, I'd spoken to Daryl, because he'd said that he wanted to come to the funeral, and I asked him to ask any of the lads in the house if they wanted to come too.

He said "Well, they might be a bit strange, and they might shout or something." I said that I didn't care, they were Edward's last friends. If they wanted to come, I wanted to see them there. And they did come and they didn't shout out, they didn't....They were a scruffy little bunch *(laughs)* but they were there. We...we played, ' Who Wants To Live Forever' Edward liked Queen, he loved Queen. 'Who Wants To Live Forever' seemed the right song for that occasion. We also played another one...there's an American singer who wrote some songs for her husband when he was dying of cancer. There was one song in there, that whenever I heard it, it made me cry and....I listen to it now when I need to cry. It summed up my feelings exactly then, of how I felt. The chorus is something like 'Only you know how I feel', which I thought 'that's what Edward knew', he knew how I felt. We played that. We read out things. Richard had written something about Edward, the person he was, and he read that out. James read a couple of Edward's poems, which he found quite hard to do and he wasn't sure if he would be able to do it but he managed. Nigel read a couple of Edward's poems, one of them was quite a funny one.

He said, when he got up there, 'If Ed could see me now, dressed in my suit with my hair cut' – because Nigel had had his hair cut as well – he said 'he'd be laughing' *(laughs)*. And I'd found a diary of Edward's, he'd kept a diary from the age of 9 to the age of 12, when he first started the prep school, until basically he left. There was all sorts of things in it. Some quite funny things; funny drawings, all sorts of stuff. There was a bit when he... he'd given marks to his old school and his new school and he'd written "I give my old school 9/20 and my new school 19/20" and then some weeks later he changed that round and he gave his new school something like 10/20 and his old school 18/20 or something, because he'd had to do a dictation and spelling test and he hadn't done that at his old school *(laughs)*. Yes there were some lovely bits in it. Afterwards when I was standing at the door saying goodbye to people, one of the teachers came up and said "I'm really sorry my dear" she said, "but I'm the one that got our school the bad marks, I gave him his dictation".

There were so many people that came; old school friends, a couple of boys who Edward had been at playgroup with and had known all through his childhood. A sister of one of them came, and she came up to me and said 'I'm here for Chris because Chris is too upset to come' she said 'but when you've got his ashes and you know where they are, can you let me know because he wants to go there on his own'.

Edward's friend, Henry, who we went to America with and who I used to take up to London with Ed, well he came up to me as he was going, and he said 'Joy, can I come round and see you?'.

I said "Yes, that would be nice Henry", and he actually came round and he spent the afternoon with me. Just talking about Edward and talking about things. I thought that was really nice of him because it must have been quite a hard thing for him to do. I really appreciated it. That he, sort of, that he spared me that time to come and talk to me. They... they were all nice kids. When we got back here after the funeral, we went into the pub and the guy in the pub just brought out a load of snacks and things *(laughs)*. He suddenly came out and put them on the table – all the family were there – he just said "There you are" and yeah, it's sort of... you don't sort of realise how good people are, and how kind they are. All the people that turned up at the funeral, sort of neighbours and people that had moved away from the village and read about it and just came along.

I'm different to how I used to be. I used to be a lot more outgoing. Now I have to make myself go out. If I had my way, I'd probably stay in all the time and just potter round the garden and do things. I do try make myself go out. I was meant to be going over to a friend's, who's a potter, ages ago to make a tile in memory of Edward and I still haven't been able to get myself to go and do it. Not that I don't want to do it – it's the effort. Having to make myself go to the workshop and do it. Not because...I know that she would be fine and be understanding and she'd accept me if I cried or whatever – it's the effort. I feel comfortable here, at home. The effort of going out is too much. I find it hard going to work, in fact I'm retiring in May. I've had so much depression and time off, it's not fair on them, on work. Nigel said recently that he realises it's not doing me any good working. Some people go to work and do things and it's good for them. For me it isn't and at the moment, because doing the job I do - in education - I'm actually dealing with young men who were born in 1980...and I find that hard. Especially when some of them remind me of Edward, either with a mannerism or something they say, or a figure of speech. Not all of them but some of them. I find that hard.

I'm having treatment for post traumatic stress. I have flashbacks and things. I don't always sleep. I still can't go to Reading really – it's an effort to go and I avoid Reading Station. It's just something I can't do at the moment. And I used to do a lot of entertaining. I used to organise parties and have people round. I find that hard. I think about it, I think 'oh, I haven't seen so and so for ages, I'll ask them over and we'll have a meal', but I can't actually do it. Couples used to come over and we'd have an ordinary sort of evening but I find that very hard to do now. Equally I find it hard, if people ask if we want to go somewhere. I have to psych myself up to do it. I do it because I know it's good for me and I know it's not fair on Nigel to...not do it. And I think not to do it wouldn't do me any good. But I do have to force myself. I don't sleep well. I appear to cope. At all levels I appear to be coping, but as soon as something comes up outside the norm...I fall to pieces. I can't cope with anything else coming in at me. Just everyday things. So it's done quite a bit of damage.

I see the damage in my other children too. Emma is suffering from quite bad depression and she's just about to get some trauma treatment. She can't cry. Whatever happens, she can't cry and they've said to her that's a strong sign of a traumatic, of something traumatic happening to her. James, on the other hand, avoids everything. He...he doesn't want to listen to any music...or anything that reminds him of Edward...and he doesn't really want to talk about Edward. When he does, he really gets upset...I mean, he sobs. His wife's expecting a baby soon, so we're hoping that's going to be, you know, a new life in the family and something positive happening. We're all looking forward to that. I think James more than anybody. He's been wanting a child ever since this happened to Edward.

In the September, when Edward came out of hospital, when he was quite well and he started college again, the week when he was staying here, he suddenly said

'Do you think I'll ever be normal Mum?',

I said 'Edward, there is hope. They have said so. In a few years time, if you continue taking your medication and you stay away from cannabis. There's a lot of hope that things will be ok. I said '25-30 seems to be the crucial age, it's not that long now, you're 20 and it will go quite quick'.

And he said 'I hope I so'. I… I really believed that that could happen. I'd actually spoken to somebody who'd had similar experiences, what they call psychotic experiences, and who'd been in a psychiatric hospital and things.

He said to me 'Don't let him down, you're his parent, be there, even if it feels like he doesn't want you. My parent's were always there for me', and that man, he's fine now. He must be in his sort of late 40's, early 50's…I wish that could have happened for Edward.

Printed in the United Kingdom
by Lightning Source UK Ltd.
106586UKS00001B/40-129

9 781904 697695